COPING WITH HEARTBURN AND REFLUX

DR TOM SMITH has been writing full-time since 1977, after spending six years in general practice and seven years in medical research. He writes the 'Doctor, Doctor' column in the *Guardian* on Saturdays, and also has columns in the *Bradford Telegraph and Argus*, the *Lancashire Telegraph*, the *Carrick Gazette* and the *Galloway Gazette*. He has written two humorous books, *Doctor Have You Got A Minute?* and *A Seaside Practice*, both published by Short Books. His other books for Sheldon Press include *Heart Attacks: Prevent and Survive, Living with Alzheimer's Disease, Coping Successfully with Prostate Cancer, Overcoming Back Pain, Coping with Bowel Cancer* and *Skin Cancer: Prevent and Survive*.

Overcoming Common Problems Series

Selected titles

A full list of titles is available from Sheldon Press,
36 Causton Street, London SW1P 4ST and on our website at
www.sheldonpress.co.uk

Assertiveness: Step by Step
Dr Windy Dryden and Daniel Constantinou

Breaking Free
Carolyn Ainscough and Kay Toon

Calm Down
Paul Hauck

Cataract: What You Need to Know
Mark Watts

Cider Vinegar
Margaret Hills

Comfort for Depression
Janet Horwood

Confidence Works
Gladeana McMahon

Coping Successfully with Pain
Neville Shone

Coping Successfully with Panic Attacks
Shirley Trickett

Coping Successfully with Period Problems
Mary-Claire Mason

Coping Successfully with Prostate Cancer
Dr Tom Smith

Coping Successfully with Ulcerative Colitis
Peter Cartwright

Coping Successfully with Your Hiatus Hernia
Dr Tom Smith

Coping Successfully with Your Irritable Bowel
Rosemary Nicol

Coping with Alopecia
Dr Nigel Hunt and Dr Sue McHale

Coping with Age-related Memory Loss
Dr Tom Smith

Coping with Blushing
Dr Robert Edelmann

Coping with Bowel Cancer
Dr Tom Smith

Coping with Brain Injury
Maggie Rich

Coping with Candida
Shirley Trickett

Coping with Chemotherapy
Dr Terry Priestman

Coping with Childhood Allergies
Jill Eckersley

Coping with Childhood Asthma
Jill Eckersley

Coping with Chronic Fatigue
Trudie Chalder

Coping with Coeliac Disease
Karen Brody

Coping with Cystitis
Caroline Clayton

Coping with Depression and Elation
Patrick McKeon

Coping with Down's Syndrome
Fiona Marshall

Coping with Dyspraxia
Jill Eckersley

Coping with Eating Disorders and Body Image
Christine Craggs-Hinton

Coping with Eczema
Dr Robert Youngson

Coping with Endometriosis
Jo Mears

Coping with Epilepsy
Fiona Marshall and Dr Pamela Crawford

Coping with Gout
Christine Craggs-Hinton

Coping with Hearing Loss
Christine Craggs-Hinton

Coping with Heartburn and Reflux
Dr Tom Smith

Coping with Incontinence
Dr Joan Gomez

Coping with Macular Degeneration
Dr Patricia Gilbert

Overcoming Common Problems Series

Coping with the Menopause
Janet Horwood

Coping with a Mid-life Crisis
Derek Milne

Coping with Polycystic Ovary Syndrome
Christine Craggs-Hinton

Coping with Postnatal Depression
Sandra L. Wheatley

Coping with SAD
Fiona Marshall and Peter Cheevers

Coping with Snoring and Sleep Apnoea
Jill Eckersley

Coping with a Stressed Nervous System
Dr Kenneth Hambly and Alice Muir

Coping with Strokes
Dr Tom Smith

Coping with Suicide
Maggie Helen

Coping with Thyroid Problems
Dr Joan Gomez

Depressive Illness
Dr Tim Cantopher

Eating for a Healthy Heart
Robert Povey, Jacqui Morrell and Rachel Povey

Effortless Exercise
Dr Caroline Shreeve

Fertility
Julie Reid

Free Your Life from Fear
Jenny Hare

Getting a Good Night's Sleep
Fiona Johnston

Heal the Hurt: How to Forgive and Move On
Dr Ann Macaskill

Help Your Child Get Fit Not Fat
Jan Hurst and Sue Hubberstey

Helping Children Cope with Anxiety
Jill Eckersley

Helping Children Cope with Change and Loss
Rosemary Wells

How to Approach Death
Julia Tugendhat

How to Be a Healthy Weight
Philippa Pigache

How to Be Your Own Best Friend
Dr Paul Hauck

How to Beat Pain
Christine Craggs-Hinton

How to Cope with Bulimia
Dr Joan Gomez

How to Cope with Difficult People
Alan Houel and Christian Godefroy

How to Improve Your Confidence
Dr Kenneth Hambly

How to Keep Your Cholesterol in Check
Dr Robert Povey

How to Make Life Happen
Gladeana McMahon

How to Stick to a Diet
Deborah Steinberg and Dr Windy Dryden

How to Stop Worrying
Dr Frank Tallis

How to Succeed in Psychometric Tests
David Cohen

How to Talk to Your Child
Penny Oates

Hysterectomy
Suzie Hayman

Is HRT Right for You?
Dr Anne MacGregor

Letting Go of Anxiety and Depression
Dr Windy Dryden

Living with Alzheimer's Disease
Dr Tom Smith

Living with Asperger Syndrome
Dr Joan Gomez

Living with Asthma
Dr Robert Youngson

Living with Autism
Fiona Marshall

Living with Crohn's Disease
Dr Joan Gomez

Living with Fibromyalgia
Christine Craggs-Hinton

Living with Food Intolerance
Alex Gazzola

Living with Grief
Dr Tony Lake

Living with Heart Failure
Susan Elliot-Wright

Living with Hughes Syndrome
Triona Holden

Overcoming Common Problems Series

Overcoming Common Problems

Coping with Heartburn and Reflux

Dr Tom Smith

sheldon **PRESS**

First published in Great Britain in 2005
Sheldon Press
36 Causton Street
London SW1P 4ST

The author and publisher have made every effort to ensure that the external website
and email addresses included in this book are correct and up to date at the time of
going to press. The author and publisher are not responsible for the content, quality
or continuing accessibility of the sites.

British Library Cataloguing-in-Publication Data

A catalogue record for this book is available from the British Library

ISBN 978–0–85969–953–2

3 5 7 9 10 8 6 4 2

Typeset by Deltatype Limited, Birkenhead, Merseyside
Printed in Great Britain by
Ashford Colour Press

Printed on paper produced from sustainable forests

Contents

Introduction

It struck me, a few pages into writing this book, which was originally entitled *Coping with GORD*, that it could be a difficult title. How many people browsing through, say, the health section of a bookshop would know what GORD is about? When I asked patients in my surgery if they knew what GORD meant, I received some funny answers, from the religious to the rude. Regular heartburn sufferers, on the other hand, were in no doubt as to what it meant. This book is for them, but for the many people with heartburn to whom GORD is a new concept, it was re-named *Coping with Heartburn and Reflux*. However, throughout the book, the term GORD will be used.

GORD stands for gastro-oesophageal reflux disease (in the USA it is called GERD because the Americans omit the 'o' from the word 'oesophagus'). In plain speak, GORD is the cause of heartburn – a symptom that almost everyone has had at some time in their lives. It also includes symptoms of upper abdominal pain and discomfort which, like the heartburn, are caused by acid and pepsin being forced upwards from the stomach through the diaphragm into the lower oesophagus, which, unlike the stomach, is not protected against acid and pepsin. The oesophagus becomes irritated and inflamed, and sometimes even ulcerated and digested by them. So the symptoms range from the relatively minor, to the major ones of eventual bleeding, perforation and even cancerous changes.

GORD is very common and getting more common. Indeed, a generation ago, there would not have been the interest in reflux disease that there is now. This new awareness is largely because of two developments in our society – our much-publicized obesity epidemic and our frenetic lifestyles.

Being overweight – specifically being apple-shaped (explained on p.3) – means that there are large amounts of fat within the abdomen. This results in there being less room for the organs inside the abdomen, and therefore more pressure upon them. There is only one way for the pressure on the stomach to be relieved – upwards through the diaphragm. Hence the squirting of stomach contents up into the oesophagus (especially when bending down or lying flat), and even the formation of hernias, in which parts of the stomach are pushed into the chest. (That's why losing weight is one of the single most effective measures you can take against GORD.)

A frenetic lifestyle – snatching meals on the hoof – means that there are plenty of hours in the day in which the stomach secretes acid and pepsin (a protein-digesting enzyme) into its cavity, but has no food to digest. This can erode both the stomach wall and the oesophagus above it.

So modern man and woman have a two-pronged attack upon them, and it is no wonder that in my surgeries in the west of Scotland I see roughly one person in every other appointments session with the symptoms of reflux disease. That extrapolated to the whole country is a very high proportion of the population – many millions. But they are only the tip of the iceberg – most people with heartburn treat themselves, and never bother to see their doctor.

This book is about GORD: how it arises, how it affects you, how it is investigated, and how it can be treated or even cured. It is for everyone with GORD who has to cope with heartburn and its related symptoms, and its consequences and complications.

Thankfully, it is a very optimistic book, because heartburn, of all 'digestive' problems, is the most easily treated. Provided you obey the rules and follow the appropriate advice on lifestyle and treatments, you can abolish it from your life.

Heartburn is not the whole story of GORD, though. If you have GORD you probably experience other symptoms that are just as annoying as heartburn. You may get fluid rising from your stomach into your mouth. That may be either 'acid brash', in which the fluid contains acid and bile, and tastes sour or bitter. Or it may be 'waterbrash', in which the mouth fills up with excess saliva. You may find it difficult and painful to swallow solid foods, no matter how well you have chewed them. You may have constant or repeated pains in the centre of the chest or upper abdomen – 'indigestion' or 'dyspepsia' – that can accompany or alternate with the heartburn. Lying flat or bending over may bring on the pain or make it worse. You may learn to avoid specific foods that seem to initiate pain. Eating too much at a time can also do it: you may already have started to eat smaller meals more often than before, in an attempt to prevent the symptoms.

Almost certainly you are used to taking anti-indigestion remedies, such as antacids or acid-suppressants. There are hundreds of proprietary medicines for GORD, and your pharmacist will probably have advised you on them and what they do. Yet still you are battling on, wondering if there is anything more you can do to help yourself.

This book is for people like you. It explains what GORD is, why it produces such pain and discomfort, and what you can do – in lifestyle changes, in eating healthily, and in medicines you can take – to become free of it and its complications. It also guides you on when you have to take things further, and how the doctors will investigate GORD to eliminate more serious illnesses or to find out whether or not you have a hiatus hernia that may need surgery to correct it. It explains what hiatus hernia is, and how it is operated on today.

Once you know the underlying cause of your symptoms, you will find it easier to cope with them and to comply with your doctor's advice. The fundamental problem in GORD is that your stomach is 'squirting' acid up into the oesophagus. Your stomach wall is resistant to acid attack, but your oesophagus is not – and that's what causes the pain. The first few chapters in this book explain why and how this happens: the rest of the book explains how we try to reverse the process and protect your oesophagus from further acid attack. First, though, you may recognize yourself in one of the case histories described in Chapter 1.

1
Some fellow sufferers

John's story
John was 60 before he had any problems with his digestion. He worked on a mixed farm of beef and dairy cattle, and the daily exercise kept him fit and slim. At 60, though, he started to take things more easily, leaving a lot of the physical work to his son and a farmhand. He began to enjoy life more, which meant relaxing more, and continuing to eat his hearty meals.

Not surprisingly, for the first time in his life John put on weight, so that within a year of his semi-retirement he was 2 stone (around 15 kilograms) heavier. That in itself didn't bother him too much, but the heartburn that came along with it became a problem. He first noticed it on the odd mornings when he helped out his son with the milking, which meant bending over to fix up the machine tubes to the cows' teats and hosing down the milking parlour afterwards.

It started as a pain in the centre of his chest that burned rather than ached. It was often accompanied by a sour taste in the mouth, and he could feel fluid rushing upwards in his throat. Sometimes it made him wheeze and gasp. He had never had asthma or any sort of chest problem before, so this worried him. He took antacids (soft chewable ones) for his heartburn, but they didn't have an as immediate effect on his wheezing as they did on his pain.

John wasn't one to go to his doctor for advice, for two reasons. Having enjoyed rude health all his life, he thought he should be able to sort for himself little things like indigestion and a wheeze. The second reason was that his doctor was his golfing partner, and he didn't like the thought of taking up his friend's time with such a trivial complaint. He was the classic example of why you shouldn't make a good friend of your doctor.

Then, one night, about an hour after going to bed after a very sociable evening of dinner and drinks, he woke with really severe heartburn and was unable to breathe. He had this burning pain in his chest and could hardly breathe out. Breathing in wasn't nearly so difficult, but he felt that with each breath he was expanding his distended chest even more, and that if he continued he might burst. He was, understandably, beginning to panic.

His wife, Anne, phoned the out-of-hours service, and the nurse on the other end of the phone quickly realized that she was dealing with an acute attack of asthma. She promised to send the emergency doctor straight round. He was there in ten minutes, and was able to ease the breathing quickly with an inhaler and an injection of hydrocortisone. However, the puzzle remained. Why did he suddenly start to have asthma at his time of life?

The next morning he saw his own doctor at the surgery. It turned out that he was even heavier than he had thought. He was now 3 stone heavier than his working weight – and, at 16 stone, he was now classifiable as obese. His blood pressure was higher, and he still was a little breathless.

His doctor read the notes of the emergency doctor from the previous evening, and noted that his breathlessness and his heartburn usually came on when he was lying down in bed. He had started to use three pillows at night, because this seemed to prevent both the 'indigestion' and the breathlessness.

The pain in the chest worried his doctor, so he arranged for a resting and exercise electrocardiogram (ECG) and a plain chest X-ray. He also asked John to blow into a 'peak flow' meter to check on his lung function. Peak flow – the maximum speed with which after a deep breath you can blow the air out of your lungs – is a measure of how elastic your lungs are. It is reduced in asthma and in chronic obstructive lung disease (what used to be called chronic bronchitis). As John had never smoked, his doctor ruled out the last diagnosis, but he wondered whether the asthma from the previous night was still lingering the next morning.

The results were encouraging. The ECGs were normal: there was no evidence of angina (which would have shown up on the exercise ECG). The peak flow was 580 litres per minute, well above the figure in active asthma or chronic lung disease. So there had to be another reason for the chest pain and the occasional wheeze.

The clue for the doctor lay in the history of burning in the centre of the chest that was eased by antacids. Could John have GORD – gastro-oesophageal reflux disease? This would explain the burning sensation, the discomfort when lying down, and the asthma. If acid is regurgitated into the throat and some of it –

even a minute quantity – is then breathed into the lungs, they can react to the irritant by narrowing. That leads to an acute breathlessness that is indistinguishable from asthma.

The fact that the burning came on most acutely when John lay down in bed or when he bent over to tend his garden or pick up his golf ball was another clue. When we are upright, gravity keeps the stomach acid where it should be – in the stomach below the diaphragm. When we bend over, the contents of the abdomen are compressed in the space between the lower ribs and the pelvis. If the stomach is surrounded by fat, then the space around it is compressed even more. The extra pressure on the stomach can cause it to squirt its contents of acid and digestive juice (a substance called pepsin) upwards into the oesophagus, in the chest. The oesophagus, unlike the stomach, can't tolerate contact with acid or pepsin, and complains about it with the burning pain.

The answer to John's problems was clear and logical. He was an 'apple' in terms of his body shape. That is, he had the particular form of obesity in which the extra weight gathered mostly around his abdomen. He had a big stomach, and relatively less obese buttocks and hips. The opposite of an apple, in terms of obesity, is a 'pear'. Pear-shaped fat people put their weight on around the hips and buttocks, rather than round their stomachs. Weight for weight, pears have fewer problems with heartburn than apples.

So the first step for John was to have his problem explained, and then to pay close attention to how he could help himself solve it. It wasn't just a matter of using antacids, although they certainly worked in the short term. John had to pay serious attention to losing the extra weight. That meant much more exercise and eating less.

Being a farmer, John wasn't in the habit of doing exercise for the sake of it. The treadmill in the gym was not for him. He enjoyed his weekly game of golf with his friends, but that was played at a leisurely pace, and the benefit he got from it was nullified by the beer in the clubhouse afterwards.

He and Anne decided to tackle the problem in two ways. They would start walking together: there were plenty of country walks they had always wanted to do, but had never taken the time.

Anne also planned their meals so that they were less fattening. Now that she and John were retired, they had slipped into the habit of eating their meals on trays while sitting on the sofa in front of the television. So they went back to their traditional meals at the table, taking their time over them, and talking about the day's events as they did so. They found that they took longer to eat their food when doing so, and that their hunger abated before they ate too much. They began to eat less, but still enjoyed their food. It didn't seem like a diet to them, but John lost a pound or two each week. That became 1 stone in two months and 3 stone within five months. By then, his heartburn had all but disappeared, and they both felt much better as a result of their new lifestyle.

That wasn't all. Because John had put on weight in that particular 'apple' pattern, his doctor gave him a full heart check. 'Apples' are at a higher risk of a stroke or heart attack than 'pears', or than people of normal shape, and they tend to have high levels of lipids (fats, cholesterol) in their blood. John's total cholesterol was initially high, at 7.7 mmol/litre. At that level, his doctor could have prescribed for him a 'statin' drug to lower it, but he decided to wait to see if the new lifestyle would bring it down first.

After two months, the total cholesterol level had fallen to 5.1 mmol/litre, giving independent evidence that John and Anne had been keeping to the healthy lifestyle guidelines. Even more important, John's total cholesterol/HDL ratio (a measure of how much of his fat was of the 'good' type that protects the artery walls against clots) was well below the critical level of 4.5. His doctor decided not to give him a statin, but instead to wait and see how well he continued to be before reconsidering.

Two years from the first consultation, John is down to 12 stone – the normal weight for his height – and feeling well. His GORD has gone. If he continues like this, it won't come back.

Joanna's story

Joanna was a busy editor of a woman's journal. At 30-something she lived life in the fast lane. She commuted from a north London suburb by tube every morning, getting into the office just before 8.30 a.m., and her day was hectic from then until she left, nearer 6 p.m. than 5 p.m., every evening. She grabbed a coffee and a slice of toast on the way out of the house for breakfast, grabbed a sandwich and another coffee for lunch, and most evenings she heated up a ready meal in the microwave, because she was too tired to cook for herself. Her partner Geoff was away on those evenings, commuting around Europe. When at home, he cooked for her. She loved the evenings when he had a meal ready, and they could relax together over home cooking and a glass of red wine.

Frankly, Joanna hadn't thought about her own health for years, even though her life revolved around producing a women's magazine every week, many of whose pages were devoted to the readers' health.

Consequently, she was thinner than she should have been – all that energy used every day, no time to replace it with food, plus many cups of black coffee – and without noticing it she continued to lose a few pounds every month. She was definitely not anorexic – she had a good appetite. She just didn't take the time to eat.

Then she started to have heartburn. It hit her around noon. At first, she took the pain as a signal that she needed to eat something, and took a few minutes off to devour a sandwich or a quick gulp of milk. That worked for a time, but the heartburn became more persistent, and began to interfere with the smooth running of her daily schedule. Chewy antacid tablets became a part of her daily routine. They helped for a while, too, but she soon realized that she had become dependent upon them, and that this wasn't healthy.

At last she talked to the journal's doctor columnist. She was too busy to go to her own doctor's surgery, which of course was miles away from the office, and closed by the time she was back home. It's not always a good idea to turn to a business colleague and friend for medical help, but just this once it was. The doctor went through Joanna's schedule in detail, and was horrified by it. She laid down the law about taking time to eat meals, and what meals she should eat. Joanna's food intake on most days was far too low for her physical and mental activities. Just as bad, she was bolting her food in a space of a few minutes snatched between appointments, meetings and frenetic efforts to meet publishing deadlines. At no time in the week (except on the evenings when she ate at home with Geoff) did she ever stop to eat a leisurely meal and rest afterwards.

Luckily, her columnist colleague was not only a caring doctor, but a good friend. The two sat down together and, over an hour or so, they discussed the reasons for her heartburn, how it was the outward symptom of several problems in her lifestyle, and how they could be resolved. In fact, the contents of the rest of this book could be seen as the range of subjects that were covered in that conversation, and in their subsequent regular discussions over the next few months.

Joanna was persuaded to slow her life down. She was asked to rise a little earlier in the weekday mornings, so that she could take some time over breakfast. Milky tea or coffee, some fruit juice, perhaps a cereal and some toast, butter and marmalade, eaten slowly over 20 minutes to half an hour, was the first rule of her day.

As the boss, she didn't always have to prove herself to her staff by arriving first in the office in the mornings. She agreed to take a later train, arrive around 9 a.m., settle into her chair, look over the day's mail, perhaps read a paper relevant to her job, and not schedule her first meeting until at least 10 a.m. From then on she could work as hard as she wished, with the strict proviso that the lunch hour was sacrosanct: a bowl of soup and a sandwich, perhaps a glass of milk or juice, eaten and drunk slowly, in the company of friends, with discussions on work ruled out. Only after the lunch hour was she to get back to work. At 5.30 p.m. at the latest, she was to pack up and go home. If all the work wasn't finished by then, she could take what she could home with her, again with the proviso that it wasn't to be opened until she had eaten her evening meal. She was asked to spend a little time in the kitchen herself, if possible, cooking easy meals for one or two, rather than ordering in a pizza.

At first she couldn't believe this advice. How could she possibly work at a slower pace, she thought, when it took her all her working time just to keep up with what she had to do? The idea was preposterous. That was when she was given the ultimatum. Either you do this, her doctor friend told her, or your health will break down – and then there will be no work to do at all.

Joanna realized that she had no choice, and tried the new regime. The walls didn't fall down when she started getting in to the office a little later. Her staff were surprised at first, but were secretly pleased that they could work peacefully and productively for a while before the whirlwind arrived. Not only that, the whirlwind had turned into a zephyr. The work still seemed to get done. The atmosphere was less fraught, and efficiency actually rose. Decisions were made faster and with more thought. The heartburn disappeared.

Joanna started to gain a little weight – just enough to look a normal shape again. She was no longer a copy of the elongated models in her magazine, and she was feeling better again. The chewable antacids were stopped, and her health improved. Although her doctor friend asked her to see her own doctor, she didn't feel the need, as her heartburn had gone. She was warned, however, that it might well return if she again put herself into a state of physical stress, and that if it did she might need more medical help.

To date, three years later, she has had no further heartburn. The magazine is going from strength to strength. However, she does have a PA who does a lot of the running around and the worrying for her. It's odd, but her PA is now getting heartburn!

Lynne's story
Lynne was 52 when she first visited her doctor. Since her children had left home and she had less to do, she had put on several stones in weight. She accepted she had a matronly figure: a more blunt description would be that she was fat. She was 5 feet 3 inches tall (1.6 metres) and weighed over 12 stone (75 kilograms).

About four years before she had started to have an ache – she described it later as 'like cramp' – in the centre of her chest that came on shortly after a snack, a meal, or even after a cup of tea. It was often linked to a sour taste, and both the pain and the taste could also be brought on by her bending over – say, to pick something up – or by the act of sitting down on her couch in the evenings.

She assumed that this was to do with her increased weight, and with the fact that she had started to wear a support girdle, and that all her doctor would say would be to tell her to lose weight. (She was probably correct about that.) So she began to treat herself by taking antacids: her favourites were Rennies.

For the first few months the antacids always eased her symptoms, quickly and efficiently. But the effect didn't last, and she soon needed to take the antacids every day, the pain lasted longer, came on more often, and seemed to be spreading further up into her chest – even into her throat. To ease it she started to drink a lot of milk and eat digestive biscuits, which did nothing for her weight problems.

The character of her pain then changed. It was now definitely a burning sensation that she could clearly define as a vertical line going from the throat to the lower margin of the ribs in the centre of her chest. It was clear to her now that she had heartburn.

Even that did not take her to her doctor. She assumed that heartburn is a common complaint, to be dealt with by over-the-counter medicines. She rang the changes on a series of different antacids – tablets, gels and liquids – and continued to wire into the dairy products.

Eventually she was forced to visit her doctor as a result of two further developments. The first was a persistent dull ache in the centre of her chest that never seemed to leave her. It sometimes woke her from sleep in the early hours. The second was that the sour taste in her mouth was becoming worse. When she was lying down at night, her mouth could suddenly fill up with a sour, watery material, that seemed to be welling up from her stomach. Once or twice she almost choked on it. She could no longer lie flat in bed. Lying on her right side in particular brought on this symptom (which she later was told was 'acid brash'). Then one night she woke up, terrified, from a deep sleep because her mouth was full of semi-digested milk. She felt she was drowning in it.

Next morning she saw her doctor, who didn't take long to make the diagnosis from the history alone. Lynne had a hiatus hernia, and it had progressed to quite a large one over the years in which she had had symptoms. He wished, of course, that she had come to him sooner, but didn't in any way blame her. He had a long discussion about what might have to be done for her, and discussed ways in which she could help herself to lose weight and to prevent the symptoms. He also started her on a drug to stop her stomach acid production – a 'proton pump inhibitor' – to try to prevent any further damage to her oesophagus and stop the cycle of pain. Why he did this is explained later in the chapters on treatment.

Since that first visit, Lynne has lost more than 2 stone of her extra 4 stone, and is feeling much better. She has had keyhole surgery to repair her hiatus hernia, and no longer has the heartburn or acid brash. She still gets occasional 'indigestion' when she fills her stomach too full, but she is much happier generally. She has got used to avoiding lying flat at night, and still sleeps on three or four pillows.

Harry's story

Harry was a schoolteacher who had no time for doctors. He had always looked after himself very well without them, and didn't see why he couldn't continue with that. Now 52, for the previous 20 years he had treated himself for mild heartburn. It was always worse just after a meal, which for Harry – who was single and had never bothered much with the niceties of cooking – was usually a fry-up.

Harry always kept a bottle of his favourite antacid mixture beside the kitchen sink, and a day wouldn't pass without him taking a swig or two from it. He was partial to a malt whisky, neat with just one cube of ice, in the evenings, while marking his pupils' work, but in recent months that had brought on the heartburn too. Even a glass of white wine gave him some discomfort, so he added anti-indigestion tablets to his mixture. The doses of medicine and tablets together mounted, month by month, as the symptoms gradually worsened.

Although he knew he was not controlling his pain as well as he might, Harry still didn't go to his doctor. It needed an emergency to force him to seek help. He woke up one morning feeling dizzy and faint. He staggered to the toilet, where he passed a motion that was the colour and consistency of warm tar. He was shivering, yet drenched in sweat. He dialled the emergency number.

It was fortunate that he did, because a black stool is a sign of bleeding. He was bleeding from an ulcer in the lowest third of his oesophagus. Over the years his oesophagus had become chronically inflamed from the upward flow of acid from his stomach. The inflammation had eventually eroded into a blood vessel. He had been on a knife-edge for many months, and was in serious danger of dying from a massive internal bleed.

Harry survived. The paramedics who arrived within a few minutes of his call had a drip into a vein in his arm within seconds and poured fluids through it to replace the blood volume that he had lost into his gut with the bleed. He was already feeling better by the time he arrived in hospital, where he received a blood transfusion and drugs to stop the bleeding and heal his oesophagus.

His lifestyle has changed. He now appreciates doctors and the primary care team that have taken over his long-term health care. He has a partner who is teaching him to cook healthily, and he is learning that fry-ups are not for him.

It turned out that Harry had 'Barrett's oesophagus', a condition in which the lower part of the oesophagus is much more prone to ulceration than normal. (It is described in Chapter 3.) It is enough to state here that Barrett's oesophagus can be life-threatening. Besides causing bleeding, as in Harry's case, it can perforate – a hole can appear in the oesophagus, allowing its contents to leak into the chest, virtually digesting the lungs. Harry could have paid with his life for his self-neglect.

Susan's story

Bleeding from an inflamed oesophagus (which is called oesophagitis) isn't always as dramatic as in Harry's case.

Susan, aged 58, had known she had a hiatus hernia for years. About five years before she had had a 'flare-up' with heartburn, waterbrash and swallowing problems. It had settled after she had received medical treatment (Chapter 5 deals with the medical treatments for GORD), and after a year or so she had virtually forgotten about it. She decided that she could manage her occasional indigestion simply by buying ranitidine (the drug she had initially been prescribed) from the pharmacy, along with antacids. This was partly because she didn't want to 'waste her doctor's time', but also because it was inconvenient arranging appointments and spending time in the waiting room just to receive a prescription that had now become a routine. She was a busy woman with a household to organize, and grandchildren to look after each day while her daughter went out to work.

Susan still had the odd bout of heartburn, but chose to ignore it. Then, in January last year, her other daughter's marriage failed. Susan cared deeply for her, and offered to help out with her children as well. Now she had four small children under eight years old to look after on most days, either after playgroup or after school closed until their respective mothers were able to take over.

It was much harder than she had envisaged. The children were all little darlings, of course, but they were normal, and not always on their best behaviour. Susan found that she wasn't coping well. She was on her feet a lot, and bending over to deal with children, toys and the usual toddler disasters and squabbles a lot of the time. She became easily breathless. She started to have dizzy spells, and might even have fainted at times if she hadn't managed to sit down quickly and put her feet up. When she did rest, she could feel her heart thumping. It took what seemed to her ages to recover her breath and for her heart to stop racing. One of her daughters, arriving to collect her children, was shocked to find her in this state, and forced her to go to her doctor.

Susan's doctor took one look at her, and tested her haemoglobin level – a measurement of the oxygen-carrying red cells in the bloodstream. At 7 grams per decilitre (g/dl), it was around half the amount it should have been. She was severely anaemic.

Her story is quite a common one. Sometimes self-treatment simply 'masks' the symptoms of reflux, leaving the lower end of the oesophagus still open to erosion by the gastric juices, both acid and pepsin. The juices eat into small blood vessels, allowing them to leak small amounts of blood into the gut. Day by day the loss of blood may be so small that it does not show up in tests of the stool, but over the years it mounts up. The bone marrow, which makes new red blood cells, can't keep replacing the small daily loss, and anaemia is the inevitable result.

Anaemia may not produce any symptoms until the person is faced with an extra physical load – such as, in Susan's case, her two extra grandchildren. The extra work forced the heart to beat faster to try to keep up the flow of oxygen to the brain and her muscles, hence the symptoms of faintness, palpitations, breathlessness and weakness. But the root cause of all her symptoms was her GORD. The reflux of acid and pepsin into her oesophagus had led to the bleeding, and then to her anaemia.

Susan was first of all given a blood transfusion to restore her haemoglobin to near-normal, and a 'proton pump inhibitor' drug (explained later) to remove the acid and allow the oesophagus to heal. Her hiatus hernia was then repaired with keyhole surgery, and the source of the problem removed. She lost her heartburn and felt well for the first time in years. Now fit enough to look after her grandchildren, she was able to organize her life better, and enjoy the youngsters rather than worry about them. Her daughters, however, appreciating the strain she had been under, helped to make life better for her by taking more time off to spend with their children. All round, everyone, including the grandchildren, benefited.

Jane's story

Jane was six months into a successful and happy first pregnancy when she had her first bout of heartburn. It appeared when she lay down on her settee one afternoon, and it was accompanied by acid regurgitation into her mouth. From then on, as she grew bigger, she found she could only take a few mouthfuls of food before she felt 'full'. At night, her heartburn kept her from falling asleep, and soon woke her up again once she had got off to sleep.

The reason for her heartburn and acid regurgitation was her pregnancy. Her growing womb was filling her abdomen, and pushing her stomach up into her chest. Many women, perhaps the majority, develop this form of reflux in the last third of their pregnancies.

There was good news for Jane. Pregnancy reflux almost always stops instantaneously after the birth. In fact, it eases a lot in the final four weeks of most pregnancies as the baby's head enters the pelvis, leaving a little more room for the stomach inside the abdomen. Pregnancy reflux is also quite easily treated: Jane was asked to sit upright, even when she was resting in the afternoon with her feet up, and to use enough pillows at night to help her sleep half-sitting up. This was a great help in keeping the acid below the diaphragm, and therefore protecting her oesophagus. She was also able to take an antacid mixture approved for pregnancy, provided by her pharmacist, that eased the heartburn whenever it appeared.

Jane's heartburn eased a few days after her son was born, and she has not had it since. She could be reassured that the reflux that she had for a time would do no permanent damage to her oesophagus, and would not leave her with a hiatus hernia or a problem with her diaphragm – often a concern for mothers.

Gordon's story

GORD isn't just an illness of adults. Gordon is a beautiful, lively, little terror of a three-year-old. He is into everything, extremely active and mischievous, but is also kind and loving. In turn he is greatly loved by his parents and worshipped by his grandparents. Yet, in the first year of his life, they thought they were going to lose him. He spent most of that year strapped into a special chair to keep him upright, day and night. It took courage and patience from his parents to help him through that year. They are amazed that the restrictions they placed on him have not affected his character or his physical activity.

The problem started when he was about six weeks old. Gordon's mum became concerned when he began to vomit back his feeds when he was laid down to rest in his cot. It wasn't just a matter of being over-fed, and simply regurgitating the extra. It happened every time he was laid flat, and the amount that he brought up was a substantial proportion of his feed. He stopped putting on weight, and began to look thinner. She and the health visitor, whom she told about her fears, worried that he might have a form of obstruction in the bowel. The health visitor arranged with the doctor for Gordon to have a test feed.

One possibility when a six-week-old baby boy starts to vomit is 'pyloric stenosis', a benign overgrowth of muscle around the outflow of the stomach into the duodenum, the first part of the bowel into which the stomach empties its load of milk. As the baby is feeding, the doctor can feel with one finger the overgrowth in the upper part of the baby's abdomen, just below the ribs. It feels like a hazel-nut. A child with pyloric stenosis shoots the milk out, like a bullet from a gun, which gives rise to the name 'projectile vomiting'. It happens with the child in any position, even when upright.

Gordon's story, though, did not sound right for pyloric stenosis. The food simply flowed out of his mouth when hc was horizontal. There was no force behind it, and it didn't happen when he was kept upright after his feeds. The doctor was also disturbed to note that there were small flecks of blood in the material Gordon was bringing up. This strongly suggested 'oesophageal irritation', caused by acid rising up into the oesophagus from the stomach.

Gordon was admitted to hospital for further checks. The specialist children's X-ray team organized a barium swallow for him – amazingly, this can be done in tiny babies. It showed a hiatus hernia, with about half of his stomach in the wrong place, above his diaphragm. There was nothing to stop the flow of acid horizontally from stomach to diaphragm when he was lying flat. When he was upright, gravity prevented the upwards flow, and he had no problem with reflux.

What was to be done? It's best to avoid surgery in small babies if we can. Most early hernias and cases of reflux will sort themselves out on their own if the baby is kept upright. As the baby grows, the stomach settles into its proper place below the diaphragm, the diaphragm develops its correct muscular function, and it stops any further upwards or even horizontal flow of acid and pepsin. The irritated oesophagus heals once that happens.

So Gordon had to be kept upright for the rest of that first year of his life. There were times when this seemed cruel, but his parents made sure that the rule was rigidly obeyed. He was strapped into his chair, and grandparents or babysitters with soft hearts were strictly warned about keeping him in that upright position, regardless of how much they wanted him to play freely on the carpet or elsewhere.

The treatment was a great success. Gordon stopped vomiting, devoured his food, put on the usual weight for his age, and has become a normal, healthy, lively child. At the age of three, he can lie flat at nights, and he never regurgitates his food. There is no looking back for him now.

It is important to diagnose reflux disease in a child as early as possible. The usual reason is a hiatus hernia that has arisen because the diaphragm has not developed completely, and there is a gap in it through which a portion of the stomach can slide or roll. If it isn't diagnosed early, the acid attack on the lower end of the oesophagus can leave it scarred and narrowed. This can leave the child with a 'short oesophagus', and the junction where it meets the top of the stomach can develop above the diaphragm, in the chest. This may need to be repaired using extensive surgery later in childhood or even in adulthood.

Vomiting when horizontal isn't the only symptom of reflux in a child. It may show up in a toddler, say, aged around one year, who makes peculiar writhing movements of the neck. The child's mum may worry that he or she is having a type of fit, which obviously is a great cause of anxiety. It's only when the contortions are shown to happen only when the child is trying to swallow some food that the reason for them becomes clear. The child is trying to use these movements to force food that is sticking in the oesophagus into the stomach. Such children know why they are making these movements, but aren't yet old enough to explain it to their parents.

Children who have reached this stage will have a narrowed oesophagus, and need specialist treatment, perhaps surgery, to help them swallow more easily and to ensure that their oesophagus, stomach and diaphragm develop properly. They must also be followed up until they are adults. About half of children who have these symptoms go on to have an adult-type hiatus hernia, and that has to be treated properly. Exactly how this is done is explained in Chapter 9.

Billy's story
Billy isn't the type you would normally associate with GORD – if, in fact, you can stereotype the very varied people who develop it anyway. He is a fitness fanatic. He began training at his local gym five years ago, and decided to make a career of it. So he passed exams in gym management and fitness, and became an instructor. He can now exercise as much as he likes, and delights in challenging his customers to keep up with him in his power exercises.

He has taken the fitness message seriously, and knows that on two days each week he has to rest, to allow his muscles to recover and replace their glucose stores. But one day he arrived at his doctor's surgery complaining of a pain behind his breastbone, and heartburn, with acid regurgitation in his mouth, particularly when he bent down or lay down. He also found he couldn't breathe as deeply as he used to, and was even getting breathless on routine exercise, something that was completely new, and even shocking, to him. He had had the symptoms for about a month, and they were not easing off. In fact, they were gradually worsening.

His doctor found him to be extremely fit, in very good shape, with well-formed muscles and no excess fat. Yet he was unable to take in a really deep breath, and was obviously most upset about his sudden deterioration in health. He was obviously in fear of losing his job, as well as frightened about what the symptoms meant. Did he have a serious illness?

His symptoms seemed to have started abruptly, on a particular day, out of the blue, which made his doctor curious. Could something unusual have happened to have caused it? Had he been in an accident or fallen?

Billy's face reddened at the memory. He had a habit of challenging his pupils – mostly young and middle-aged business types – to throw a medicine ball directly at his stomach, as hard as they could. The aim was to test how strong his stomach muscles were, and to compare them with others in the group. As they were friends who enjoyed relaxing together, the session ended in horseplay, with medicine balls being thrown at random. He had been hit square in the navel unexpectedly by one of the medicine balls when he was off guard, and it had winded him quite badly for a while. Billy dated the start of the symptoms from that moment. He hadn't volunteered the information as he thought that it might show him up in an unprofessional light.

His doctor wasn't at all bothered by that. Instead, he was concerned that real damage might have been done to Billy's diaphragm. A sudden rise in pressure inside the abdomen might well cause a tear in the diaphragm, and allow some of the stomach to slip up into the chest – a 'traumatic' hiatus hernia. This could easily produce the combination of heartburn, chest pain and acid regurgitation that Billy had described.

This isn't a unique story. A sharp blow on the abdomen with a blunt object may leave no external bruising, but can still damage the internal organs. Harry Houdini was killed by just the same challenge that Billy had issued. The great escapologist used to challenge people to come on to the stage and punch him as hard as they could in the stomach. He rode the punch with equanimity because he tensed his muscles before the hit. One day a young man, seeing Houdini in a restaurant, punched him hard in the stomach. Houdini didn't know the punch was coming, and his stomach muscles were relaxed. The punch ruptured his appendix, and he died a few days later of peritonitis.

Billy, happily, didn't share Houdini's fate. An X-ray showed that a fairly large proportion of his stomach had slipped into his chest through a tear in his diaphragm. He was sent to the surgeons, who repaired the tear after putting his stomach back in the abdomen where it belonged. Billy recovered well and went back to the gym to continue his career. He gave up his 'stomach wall challenge', though. He realized he had been lucky. If a loop of bowel had been full of gas at the time the medicine ball hit him, he might have ruptured that too – and that would have been altogether more serious.

Archie's story

Archie is a retired electrician. His main symptom of GORD was hiccups. They started when he was in his early fifties, and tended to come on when he was in bed, just before dropping off to sleep. He noticed that they were more likely to start if he had eaten sweets, cream or chocolate just before going to bed. He had, he said, a 'sweet tooth'. At the same time, he felt a 'discomfort' – it wasn't really a pain or burning sensation – in the top of his abdomen just below where the breastbone ends. He also spoke of a bloated feeling inside his chest, as if gases were trapped inside it. When he had this feeling he wanted to belch, but couldn't.

He assumed that he had 'indigestion' and changed his late evening eating habits, avoiding sweet things and drinking a glass of milk instead. The discomfort and bloating did ease off, and he felt better, but he still had, from time to time, hiccups at bedtime.

Archie soon found that he could relieve the hiccups by getting out of bed and walking around, or by propping himself almost upright in bed on four or five pillows. After a few nights of difficulty with sleeping in this new position, he gradually got used to it, and eventually he was sleeping well.

Much of Archie's work involved wiring houses, including re-wiring old houses. That meant he spent a lifetime crawling under floorboards. Doing that one day, at the age of 60, he suddenly developed a severe pain in the centre of his chest, felt very sick, and became cold, clammy and sweaty. A doctor was called, and he was admitted to hospital with a suspected heart attack.

Happily, the hospital tests showed that he had no heart problem but an inflamed gallbladder, full of gallstones. It was assumed that his symptoms were all due to that one problem, and he was given a course of antibiotics to remove the inflammation and booked in for 'cold surgery' to remove the gallbladder a few weeks later. This is standard practice for gallstones, and the surgery eventually was successful.

While the surgeons were operating, though, they had a routine look around inside the abdomen. They found a small hiatus hernia

17

that they felt was not serious enough to repair, so left it as it was. Archie was told about this after the operation.

Since the operation, Archie has been careful about what he does and doesn't do. He no longer has the discomfort in his upper abdomen – that was almost certainly part of his gallbladder problem. But occasionally he still gets hiccups and the bloated feeling in his chest. If he avoids bending over or eating anything after 8 p.m., he has few symptoms. Recently, eight years after the operation, he has been having the odd episode of heartburn, for which he takes a ranitidine (Zantac) tablet a day, which seems to help.

Two other changes in his life may have been of significant benefit. Now that he has retired he doesn't have to crawl around under floors, or lie on a floor with his head down a hole – both being conducive to forcing acid from the stomach into the oesophagus.

The other change is probably even more significant for his long-term health: he has stopped smoking. He smoked for 40 years and gave it up after the operation, on the strong advice of his anaesthetist, who explained what the habit was doing to his lungs. He feels much the better for stopping. Everyone, smokers included, knows how smoking harms the heart and lungs. Far fewer people, though, understand that smoking directly irritates the stomach wall as well, and increases the acidity of the stomach juices. Many smokers, like Archie, find that the act of stopping smoking is in itself enough to greatly ease their symptoms.

Having retired, he has also had the time (which he didn't before) to take up golf. Playing three or four rounds a week, he has lost over 2 stone (13 kilograms) in weight. This too has eased his symptoms: he can bend over now without precipitating discomfort or heartburn.

Archie's case carries an important message for doctors and patients alike. One in every five people with heartburn and regurgitation – the two main symptoms of GORD – has another illness that can produce similar symptoms. Among them are duodenal and stomach ulcers, gallstones and coronary heart disease. Even if a person has been proved by an X-ray or endoscopy to have a hiatus hernia that might fully explain the symptoms, it should never be assumed that any symptoms in the upper abdomen or in the centre of the chest are necessarily caused by the hernia.

If you know that you have GORD, and you develop any new symptoms, as Archie did, don't hesitate to seek advice about them. It can often be difficult to distinguish between the pain of GORD in the oesophagus and the pain of a heart attack. One thing about them is sure – an antacid will usually give fast relief to the pain of an oesophagus irritated by GORD, but it will have no effect on pain caused by a heart attack. If you don't get quick relief when you treat chest pain with an antacid, you must call for the emergency services immediately.

Mike's story

Mike was 47, a reasonably successful senior lecturer at a busy technical university, when he started to have difficulty with his voice. He noticed that, by the time he was about two-thirds through his usual hour of speaking to his students, he was becoming hoarse. He had developed a slight cough, despite being a non-smoker and having no history of asthma. He wasn't quite as fit as before, noticing that he was a bit breathless climbing hills – which was quite unusual because, as a Scottish hill enthusiast, he was a 'Munro-bagger'. He had 'bagged' more than a hundred of these 3,000-foot mountains in the Highlands in the previous ten years, and was upset at the thought that he might not be able to continue.

Things gradually worsened. The hoarseness became a permanent feature of his voice, the cough became worse and more persistent, and he began to lose weight, mainly because his appetite was not as good as it had been, and partly because it seemed to him that it took a smaller amount of food to make him feel 'full'.

As his doctor, I was worried about the combination of the hoarse voice and the loss of weight, being trained to think that I must rule out a throat cancer before all else. So my first step was to have an Ear Nose and Throat (ENT) specialist look at Mike's vocal cords. The ENT surgeon gave Mike the all-clear, but he suggested in his letter to me that Mike might have 'Cherry-Donner syndrome', a condition in which gastro-oesophageal reflux produces a hoarse voice with a cough and occasional breathlessness.

I therefore passed Mike on to a gastroenterologist with an interest in GORD, who, on endoscopy, found the reflux. Mike was put on a high dose of a proton pump inhibitor, and his hoarseness gradually subsided. He regained his appetite, started to put on weight, and could lecture again without his voice failing him. Best of all for him was that he lost his breathlessness and could continue his hill walking. I can't keep up with him!

What had made me miss the diagnosis initially was that Mike had never complained about heartburn. I hadn't heard of people who might have severe *oesophagitis* (inflammation of the oesophagus) without heartburn, as Mike had, and that threw me off the diagnostic track. So why should the breathlessness have improved? People who have repeated 'squirts' of acid rising in their oesophagus can breathe in some of this acid. It irritates the lungs, which react by producing coughs in attempts to rid the lungs of the unwanted intruder. Stomach acid in the lungs can even result in pneumonia, lung abscesses and chronic lung fibrosis, which leads to permanent breathlessness if not spotted early enough. So I was very happy that Mike's breathlessness improved. Once I heard that his cough had been due to breathing in stomach acid because of reflux, I was worried that the damage might have been permanent.

Mike gave me permission to use his case history in this book, and when I started to read more about conditions like his, I was upset that I had missed the diagnosis. I should have made it from his history, which combined hoarseness, persistent coughing and difficulties in eating with loss of weight. The medical journals show that in 6 to 10 per cent of people with a chronic cough, the cause is GORD. Mike's case is by no means rare – I failed to make the diagnosis because I did not know that. I won't make the same mistake again.

Summarizing the case histories

Reading through these case histories you will realize that GORD affects people of all ages, sizes, occupations and backgrounds, and both sexes. Each person experiences the symptoms of the illness in his or her unique way. The main symptoms, though, are heartburn, discomfort in the chest, and reflux of acid brash up into the mouth from the stomach, or the production of excess saliva as waterbrash.

Most people with GORD can control their symptoms with a

change in lifestyle, although many need drugs to help them, and a few need surgery to correct the problem (such as a hiatus hernia) that is causing their symptoms. From Chapter 3 onwards, the lifestyle changes, the medicines and the surgery will be described in more detail.

To understand why GORD causes so much distress, however, you need to know a little about the anatomy (structure) and physiology (function) of the oesophagus, the stomach and the diaphragm, and how the stomach produces and protects itself against its digestive juices. At the root of all the trouble is the fact that the oesophagus has no such protection. How, in people with GORD, we can return the oesophagus, the diaphragm and the stomach to normality is the main message of this book. If you know about that, you are well on your way to a cure.

2
The normal oesophagus, diaphragm and stomach

To understand why you have GORD you need to know about the normal workings of the oesophagus, diaphragm and stomach. The first thing to understand is the action of normal swallowing. The only part of swallowing that we are normally conscious of happens at the back of the tongue and the throat. From the moment the food and drink reach the top of the oesophagus, we are unaware of the rest of the process. Yet it is a very active one. The oesophagus is a muscular tube, and the muscles around it, along its length, co-ordinate their movements so that its contents are squeezed downwards, like emptying an inverted toothpaste tube from the base downwards to the nozzle.

Swallowing is not just the result of gravity. We transfer food towards the back of our throat using our tongue. Swallowing then becomes automatic, in that although we can feel the food slipping down towards the oesophagus we cannot stop it from doing so. It is now under the control of the 'autonomic nervous system', a network of nerves that combine to control the movements of food through the rest of the gut, without our being aware of it.

When food hits the back of the throat (the pharynx) it stimulates two muscle reflexes: one shuts off the passages back into the mouth, the back of the nose and the lungs. The other squeezes the food down into the upper part of the oesophagus. By doing this we can't inhale and swallow at the same time. Food in the lungs is a disaster that can quickly lead to death.

The oesophagus

The oesophagus is a very muscular tube. The action of the autonomic nerves causes it to contract and relax in a very controlled and co-ordinated way, so that it actively pushes solids and liquids onwards from the throat into the stomach. These ripples are called 'peristalsis'. They occur throughout the whole gut, from oesophagus to anus, and are the means by which food, and then faeces, are passed onwards. If peristalsis fails, the food simply sticks where it is lying. Liquid may trickle downwards, but solids will stay in a lump, stretching the tube walls and causing serious discomfort.

Three types of muscle contractions make up the peristaltic process:

1 Once we start to swallow, primary peristaltic waves ripple down the oesophagus, pushing food in front of them at a rate of 5 centimetres a second.
2 If the primary peristaltic waves don't manage to empty the contents of the oesophagus into the stomach, a secondary wave starts, about halfway down the oesophagus. This reinforces the primary wave, and sometimes it can be felt as an uncomfortable, almost indescribable, feeling, deep in the chest. It was a main symptom in several of the case histories in Chapter 1, and readers with GORD will almost certainly recognize it.
3 Radiologists categorize a third form of muscle contraction in the oesophagus, which they describe as 'tertiary' when they are watching the progress of barium swallow studies. They occur in one segment of oesophagus at a time. They don't appear to be involved in swallowing, and don't propel food forwards. We don't know why they appear. One suggestion is that they are a way of keeping the oesophageal muscles in tone between meals, while waiting for the next lump of food to come down.

Peristalsis is vital for transferring solid and semi-solid food from the back of the throat into the stomach. If we are upright, liquids can trickle down the oesophagus by themselves. Once we swallow a liquid, as long as there is no obstruction to its flow, it enters the stomach by gravity alone. However, peristalsis is needed to ensure that fluids won't return up from the stomach into the throat. Without it, if you swallowed a drink when lying flat, or even upside down, the drink or food would flow back into the mouth.

My colleagues and I in my year at medical school have graphic memories of being taught about swallowing. Dr Hillary Harries, one of our physiology lecturers, brought into the lecture hall a pint of beer, climbed on to the demonstration table, stood on his head facing us, then drank the beer in one go. He didn't find it difficult and didn't spill a drop. He declined to perform an encore!

So the rippling muscles of the oesophagus ensure that the passage of food and drink through it is one-way only. This is very important. If food travels in the other direction you are sick – vomiting – and you feel awful with it.

At its lower end the oesophagus passes through a hole – in Latin, this is the *hiatus* – in the diaphragm, a sheet of muscle that separates the contents of the chest from the organs in the abdomen. Below the diaphragmatic hiatus, the oesophagus becomes the upper part of the stomach. How it does so, and how the stomach and oesophagus relate to the diaphragm, are crucial to understanding GORD.

It is vital that the one-way flow of food through the oesophagus is continued when it reaches the stomach. Once in the stomach, it has to stay there for a while to allow mixture of the food with the stomach's digestive juices, and then pass forward into the duodenum, the first part of the small bowel. The stomach's digestive juices are very acid so that they can break down proteins (mainly meats and fish) into their constituent parts, before being taken up through the small bowel wall into the body. The stomach wall is largely protein, so it would digest itself if it weren't protected against its own juices.

That protection takes two forms. There are four main types of 'secreting' cells in the stomach lining. One provides the acid (hydrochloride acid) that initiates protein breakdown. Another provides the pepsin that digests the proteins even further. A third provides a thick mucus that spreads over the whole of the stomach lining to protect it from acid attack. The fourth secretes bicarbonate that neutralizes excess acid, adding more protection against self-digestion.

At the lower end of the stomach the bicarbonate secretion begins to predominate, so that the duodenum receives a mixture of semi-digested food at a much less acid level – almost neutral – than the material in the main body of the stomach. When the protective mechanisms of mucus and bicarbonate break down or are diminished, the stomach does start to self-digest, leading to ulcers – exposed areas of stomach lining that are inflamed and eroded. Stomach ulcers are usually due to a failure of the balance between the stomach's digestive secretions and its self protection mechanisms. They are often called 'peptic' ulcers because the combination of pepsin and acid is a powerful cause of erosion of the underlying stomach wall.

Understanding this balance between digestive secretions and self-protection is vital if you need to understand what is going on in GORD. If the acid and pepsin of the stomach somehow finds its way upwards into the lower oesophagus, the balance between digestion and protection has gone. The cells that line the oesophagus do not secrete a mucus protection or bicarbonate: they offer no protection at all against the acid and pepsin. So if acid and pepsin enter the oesophagus there is an immediate reaction. The cells respond with irritation and inflammation, and the brain interprets this as heartburn and pain. If the process continues for more than a few hours, ulcers form in the lower end of the oesophagus; and when they eventually heal, they may do so with scarring that can narrow it. Long exposure of the oesophagus to the stomach's secretion can eventually lead to multiple scarring, bleeding and even perforation of the oesophagus, complications that are obviously dangerous and life-threatening.

It's crucial for normal health, therefore, that we keep the stomach contents out of the oesophagus. The body tries its best to do so, using several mechanisms working together in mutual co-operation. They are the cardia, the sphincter and the diaphragm. Knowing how each of them contributes to keeping stomach juices out of the oesophagus is essential to understanding what may produce GORD.

The cardia

The last 5 centimetres or so of the oesophagus lie under the diaphragm in the abdomen (see Figure 1). The oesophagus meets the stomach at its upper right-hand surface, not quite at the top. If the stomach were a clock face, and you were looking at it from the front, the meeting of the oesophagus and the stomach (the oesophageal-stomach junction) would be at 11 o'clock.

This junction is the 'cardia'. It meets the stomach at an angle, so that food slides easily downwards from the oesophagus into the bottom 90 per cent of the stomach. It is not unlike tipping a glass to one side when you pour a fizzy drink into it, to avoid turbulence and froth. The angle should also ensure that, if there is any reverse movement of food upwards in the stomach, it passes by the entry into the oesophagus (the cardia) and ends up in the top 10 per cent of the stomach. Continuing the analogy with the clock face, that's the 12 o'clock area, or the 'fundus'.

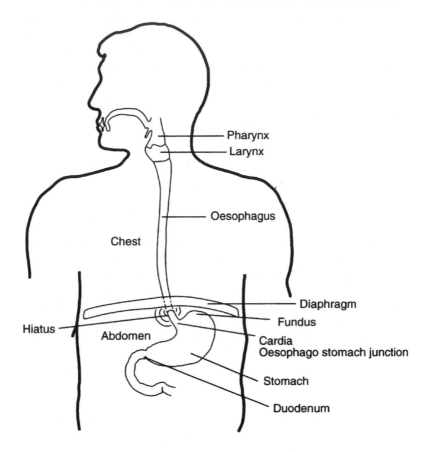

Figure 1   The normal oesophagus, diaphragm and stomach

The fundus, being the uppermost part of the stomach, is virtually an unexpanded balloon. It is a safety valve that gathers any gas that has been swallowed with food (that's why we 'burp' babies after their feeds) or produced during digestion. It normally sits neatly under the diaphragm.

The sphincter

At the cardia, just where the oesophagus becomes the stomach, there is a ring of muscle around it, within its wall. Imagine a bicycle inner tube that is semi-inflated with an elastic band around it, gripping it a little and narrowing it. Then transfer that image to the oesophagus as the inner tube, and the sphincter muscles as the elastic band. Sphincters exist at crucial areas of the gut where it is important for there to be no back-flow. The first sphincter in the line between mouth and anus is the one between the oesophagus and the stomach, at the cardia. The next is at the pylorus, where the food passes from the stomach into the duodenum. The third is where the contents of the small bowel (the ileum) enter the large bowel (the caecum), so it is called, fairly obviously, the ileo-caecal sphincter. The last is between the rectum and anus, the anal sphincter. That's the one that helps to make us sociable human beings: it allows us to refuse the natural call to pass a motion.

To return to the gastro-oesophageal sphincter. The angle at which the oesophagus meets the stomach, as mentioned above, is important in preventing reflux. However, so is the efficiency of the sphincter at the same site. It opens (in other words, the muscle of the sphincter relaxes) to let food and drink pass from oesophagus to stomach, and it closes to prevent the food flowing back from stomach to oesophagus. It is a one-way valve that normally works perfectly.

As well as the sphincter muscles themselves, there is another group of muscles that keeps this valve structure intact. These are the obliquely positioned muscles that keep the oesophagus and stomach at the appropriate angle to each other, much like a sling or hammock. Without these muscles, the angle between oesophagus and stomach would flatten out and the bottom end of the oesophagus would open in a straight line full on to the stomach. That would make back-flow very much easier.

Such back-flow pressures mount up when the stomach, full of

food, starts its job of digestion. Like the oesophagus, the stomach wall has peristaltic waves flowing through it, which propel the food from above downwards, towards the outlet at the pyloric sphincter into the duodenum. However, it is also subject to chaotic churning waves of muscle activity that are helpful in mixing the stomach contents thoroughly with the digestive juices. If the gastro-oesophageal sphincter and the oblique muscle fibres are not working properly and together, this may allow the chaotic waves to push the stomach contents backwards, up into the lower oesophagus – and this is reflux, and the start of GORD.

Abdominal pressure

Another factor, the pressure inside the abdomen, now comes into the reckoning in any understanding of GORD. The biggest difference between the cavities within the chest and the abdomen is the pressure inside them. Inside the chest the pressure is much lower than the pressure inside the abdomen. It rises further inside the abdomen when we are trying to push the stools out with defaecation, or when we exert ourselves in other ways – say, lifting a heavy weight or bending over, or digging: in fact, any activity for which we have to tense (contract) our abdominal muscles – the 'six-pack' so loved by body builders, but which the rest of us mortals hide in various degrees of fat.

A higher pressure inside the abdomen than inside the chest means that there is a constant force that tends to drive the contents of the stomach upwards. The organ that both maintains that high difference in pressure and at the same time prevents the upward movement of stomach contents is the diaphragm. If you have GORD, above all else you should understand what your diaphragm does for you.

The diaphragm

The diaphragm is a tough sheet of muscle attached in an umbrella-shaped circle around the lower margin of the ribs. Above it are the heart and lungs: below it, on the right side, is the liver, and on the left side, the spleen. Nestling up against the rear under-surface of the diaphragm on each side, near the spine, is a kidney. Under the centre of the diaphragm, towards the front, is the stomach: the fundus lying comfortably up against it. On a straight X-ray of the stomach, the gas bubble that often lies in the fundus is used by radiologists to outline the under-surface of the diaphragm.

Obviously there have to be holes in the diaphragm to allow essential tubes to pass through it between the chest and the abdomen. One, near the front, accommodates the oesophagus. Others, near the back, allow the main artery (the aorta) and vein (the inferior vena cava) to pass through. For the diaphragm to be effective in preventing upwards movement of the stomach contents, the oesophageal hole – the hiatus mentioned in the last chapter – has to be virtually pressure-tight. So there are powerful muscles in the diaphragm around the rim of the hiatus that hold it close to the oesophagus. These muscles criss-cross around the oesophagus as it passes through in the hiatus, so they are called the diaphragmatic crura. Under normal circumstances, nothing can pass between the crural edges and the outer oesophageal surface.

This arrangement of muscles around the hiatus is very useful for preventing a hernia (a piece of stomach sliding or rolling up into the chest through the hiatus). It also ensures that the external pressure around the last few centimetres of the oesophagus (the part that lies inside the abdomen) is high – at least as high as the pressure inside the rest of the abdomen.

So even if the cardia is slightly inefficient, and could possibly allow the stomach contents back up into the oesophagus, this backflow is prevented by the high external pressure exerted by the crura. They effectively keep the oesophagus collapsed until the pressure of food and peristalsis from above opens it up. This positive pressure produced by the crura on the lower end of the oesophagus is probably the most important mechanism for preventing the backflow of the stomach contents. If the cardia is pushed up into the chest cavity, as may happen with a hernia, for example, then the effect of the crura is lost, the surrounding pressure is much lower, and backflow into the oesophagus becomes the rule rather than the exception.

If you have managed to read this far without becoming confused, congratulations. You are beginning to realize that what goes on in the act of swallowing is complex, and that the flow of food downwards from the oesophagus is achieved through the combination of a series of mechanisms, any one of which could fail, leading to reflux.

To summarize the normal processes

- The oesophagus uses a series of muscular contractions to push the food down through the diaphragm.
- The crura, the muscles that form the rim of the hole (hiatus) in the diaphragm through which the oesophagus passes, by their tight fit around the oesophagus ensure that the food does not make an unwanted return upwards.
- Just below the diaphragm, the pressure on the last portion of the oesophagus reinforces that function. When there is no food in the oesophagus, the portion below the hiatus is collapsed. It only opens when food presses on it from above, to reach the cardia, the junction between the lowest part of the oesophagus and the stomach.
- At the cardia, the muscle activity in the sphincter and the oblique muscles that maintain the angle at which the oesophagus meets the stomach combine to ensure that the food enters the stomach smoothly and cannot return. It is a perfect system.
- When these things work together, we are totally unaware that all the various systems are doing their job. It is only when one (or more) of them goes wrong that we develop the symptoms of GORD.

How they may go wrong is explained in the next chapter.

3

When things go wrong –
the causes of GORD

Things, sadly, do go wrong with the mechanisms that are meant to prevent reflux, and Drs M. Ruth, I. Manson and N. Sandberg showed just how often in the *Scandinavian Journal of Gastroenterology.*[1] Their research covered northern Europe, and there's no reason to suppose that things have changed for the better, or that they are different from the British figures. They reported that, depending on the populations studied, a massive 21 to 40 per cent of the general public have heartburn in any six-to-twelve-month period. Among these people, the severity of their problems range from the most common finding of 'endoscopy-negative GORD', to, in about 8 per cent of them, oesophagitis so severe that they have ulcers and strictures (narrowings due to scarring). In between are the people who are shown by endoscopy to have an irritated and inflamed mucosa: the mucosa is the sheet of cells that line the inner surface of the oesophagus – the surface that is seen through an endoscope.

With so many people having heartburn from time to time, it's obvious that most cases can't be caused by serious structural problems in the oesophagus, diaphragm or stomach. Only a minority have, for example, a hiatus hernia to explain their symptoms. In the vast majority of cases the cause seems to be periods during which the gastro-oesophageal sphincter muscles relax, allowing upward flow of gastric juices into the lower third of the oesophagus. More than half of all those who have heartburn so often and so severely that they are referred by their GP to a gastroenterology centre have no abnormality on their endoscopy. Their mucosa looks normal. They are the people who are diagnosed as having endoscopy-negative GORD.

Being given this diagnosis is in no way to belittle the symptoms or the effect they may be having on your life. The heartburn and other symptoms of GORD are certainly bad enough, even in people with endoscopy-negative results, to make life a misery. They are just as debilitating as, say, coronary heart disease.[2] GORD is painful, can cause considerable mental stress and interfere badly with your social life.[3] The symptoms are all caused by the exposure of the oesophagus to the acid and pepsin from the stomach, and some people's oesophageal linings may be more sensitive to them than others. So, being endoscopy-negative simply means that, happily for you, the reflux has not yet damaged the cells of your oesophagus, and that you can be given medical treatment that will help you. It doesn't mean that you don't need to have the full treatment to help relieve the pain. It also means that most people with GORD do not need tests and complex investigations: they are reserved for the minority who do not respond to initial treatment, or whose GORD is so severe that the doctor expects some complication and considers that you are at extra risk.

As the case histories in Chapter 1 have shown, heartburn is not the only symptom of GORD. In fact, as with Mike, it may not be present at all. Doctors now divide cases into 'typical', 'atypical' and 'respiratory', and make the diagnosis of GORD mainly from the mixture of symptoms that the patients present to them.

Typical symptoms include, first and foremost, heartburn, defined as:

A burning feeling rising from the stomach or lower chest up towards the neck that is related to meals, lying down, stooping and straining, and is relieved by antacids.

Patients who identify with this clear definition have already diagnosed themselves. They have GORD, and they can start on treatment for it without having to wait for further tests or investigations.

Other typical symptoms include discomfort behind the breastbone, acid brash (regurgitation of acid or bile), waterbrash (excess saliva in the mouth) and pain on swallowing (medically, this is called 'odynophagia'). Patients with pain when they swallow do need urgent investigation as it may be due to severe oesophagitis with ulceration and bleeding or a stricture caused by scars from old episodes.

Atypical symptoms include pain in the centre of the chest, very similar to angina or the pain of a heart attack, pain in the upper abdomen ('epigastric' pain), and bloating, a feeling that you can experience in the chest and in the abdomen.

It is difficult for doctors and paramedic staff in emergency ambulances to differentiate initially between the chest pain of acute GORD and a heart attack, because the quality of the pain in the two cases is very similar. It's now recognized that, in chest pain emergencies, half of the patients who have normal electrocardiograms (ECGs), and no signs of coronary disease showing on angiograms, actually have acute GORD. One clue to the real diagnosis is that there is no relationship between GORD chest pain and exercise or acute mental or physical stress. Angina, on the other hand, is closely related to exercise and stress.

The respiratory symptoms include wheezing, breathlessness and cough. The Cherry-Donner syndrome (described in Chapter 1, in Mike's case) is typical of the breathing problems faced by some people with GORD. Anyone who has an unexplained cough that doesn't resolve within two or three weeks is now automatically a candidate for the diagnosis of GORD. Minute amounts of acid spilling up to the larynx (the voice box) and then breathed into the lungs is enough to produce a cough. That's especially true for non-smokers. Smokers have other strong reasons for coughing, such as chronic obstructive lung disease and lung cancer, but that's another story. A non-smoker who has a permanent cough, and has not had a previous history of asthma, is considered to have GORD until proved otherwise.

What brings on GORD?

Smoking

So what does bring on GORD? Let's go back to smoking. If you smoke, you will make your GORD worse, whether or not you develop respiratory symptoms. This is so important to understand that if you don't want to stop smoking, there's no point in reading on any further. You are a lost cause, and any treatment you have for GORD will probably be nullified by your cigarette habit. You cannot continue to smoke and expect to have your symptoms relieved. Smoking not only increases the acid production by your stomach, it will also help to relax that vital gastro-oesophageal sphincter. Worse, if you continue to smoke, you will steeply increase your chances of converting the chronic inflammation in your lower oesophagus into cancer. The sooner you give up the weed, the better your chances of your symptoms disappearing and your survival into a happy and healthy old age.

Alcohol

I'm sorry to sound a killjoy, but if you have GORD, you must also be very careful about your alcohol consumption. The neater the alcohol you drink, the more likely you are to provoke an attack of acute GORD. So, although as a Scot it pains me to write this, ease off on the spirits. Confine yourself to the odd glass of wine, preferably with meals. That's how the French approach alcohol, and it's very civilized. They have less GORD than we do.

Clothing

Not all GORD sufferers are the same. Some can tolerate coffee or fatty foods, others can't. Being overweight and eating large meals certainly cause GORD, as does pregnancy (see the case histories for typical examples). Tight clothes can put pressure on the abdomen, so that if I were writing this book a generation ago, I would have mentioned corsets. However, I'm reliably informed (by my slim wife) that women no longer squeeze into restrictive clothing – they just 'let it all hang out'. Any tight band across the middle, such as a belt, may induce reflux. I leave it to the individual woman (or man) to judge whether or not that is a factor in their GORD.

Medication

Some prescription drugs can contribute to GORD by causing the sphincter at the cardia to relax. They include the 'tricyclics' used to treat depression. They are usually easily spotted, because their generic name (seen in small print under the trade name) often ends in -amine or -ine. Among them are amitriptyline, amoxapine, clomipramine, imipramine, lofepramine, nortriptyline and trimipramine. 'Anticholinergic' or 'atropine-like' drugs prescribed to treat bowel spasms or irritable bowel syndrome can do their job only too well and relax the gastro-oesophageal sphincter, too. They include dicyclomine (also called dicycloverine), hyoscine and propantheline bromide. Atropine sulphate tablets are given on prescription but are also available over-the-counter, mainly as Actonorm powder, which is a mixture of atropine, aluminium, calcium carbonate, magnesium, sodium bicarbonate and peppermint oil. This, too, can relax the gastro-oesophageal sphincter and provoke attacks of GORD.

Another group of drugs that may cause GORD is the 'nitrates' prescribed to open the coronary arteries for people suffering from angina. Among them are glyceryl trinitrate and isosorbide trinitrate and mononitrate. If your chest pain becomes worse when taking these drugs, you either are having more serious heart pain than you thought, and should urgently see your doctor, or the pain is caused by GORD. Either way, you need help.

Some drugs directly irritate the oesophageal mucosa. They include the aspirin-like non-steroidal anti-inflammatory drugs used to treat chronic pain; potassium salts that are sometimes used in people taking drugs to lower blood pressure; and the bisphosphonates given for osteoporosis. If you are on treatment for any of these conditions, and think you may be taking one of these types of drug, you should discuss it with your doctor.

So if you have GORD and are taking drugs for other conditions, check with your doctor that your treatment is not worsening your GORD symptoms. There are always alternatives to be found if they are.

Oesophageal disorders

This part of the book would not be complete without mentioning conditions of the oesophagus that either predispose themselves, or their treatment predisposes them, to GORD.

Barrett's oesophagus

The most important of these is Barrett's oesophagus. In 1950, British surgeon N. R. Barrett wrote a paper entitled 'Chronic peptic ulcer of the oesophagus and oesophagitis'. It was published in the *British Journal of Surgery*, since when the name Barrett's oesophagus has been given to all such cases.

People with Barrett's oesophagus have two main symptoms. They have heartburn, which is usually severe, and their food tends to come back into their mouth ('regurgitation'). Even when they have not been eating, those with Barrett's find bitter gastric secretions welling up into their mouths. If the condition is not diagnosed early and treated, they develop difficulties in swallowing ('dysphagia'), and a severe 'boring' pain in the centre of the chest that can travel through to the back. The dysphagia is a sign that scarring in the oesophagus is causing it to narrow (a stricture), and that food can no longer pass through it easily. The second is a sign of an ulcer in the oesophagus. Both are serious developments that must be treated. If they are not, the next stage can be bleeding (haemorrhage) from the ulcer, or even perforation of the ulcer into the chest cavity, with all the damage that can be wrought if the lungs are exposed to the stomach's digestive juices.

In Barrett's oesophagus the flaw is in the lining of the lower end of the oesophagus. Instead of it having the usual tough, skin-like cells that line the normal oesophagus, its lining is much more like the lining of the stomach wall, with glands and other cells that are much more susceptible to acid attack, but that do not produce adequate amounts of the mucus that normal stomach cells generate to protect themselves. As the Barrett's oesophagus is also often linked to a hiatus hernia, it is repeatedly exposed to the stomach's digestive juices. The ensuing irritation and inflammation lead to the strictures and the ulcers. There are even acid-producing cells within the Barrett's tissue itself, so that it contains the mechanism of its own destruction.

Obviously people with a Barrett's oesophagus are at higher risk of serious illness than others with uncomplicated GORD. Without further tests, too, it is difficult to tell just from the symptoms alone whether the person has it or not. This is why any suspicion of Barrett's oesophagus (say if the symptoms are severe or there is constant chest pain or difficulty in swallowing) should be confirmed by endoscopy. The next chapter explains how we make the decision to go ahead with an endoscopy.

Why people have a Barrett's oesophagus in the first place is still a matter of argument among the experts. It was initially thought to be a defect that people were born with. Opinion has now swung to its being acquired after birth, although when and why is not yet known. In 22 years of studying patients with hiatus hernias, American surgeons J. Borrie and L. Goldwater found that 4.5 per cent of them had a Barrett's oesophagus. They fell into two groups: children from birth to 15 years old, and adults from 48 to 80 years old. Three times as many men as women had it, and some families had more than one member with it.

Barrett's oesophagus has been linked with cancer, but this too is a subject of controversy. There have been repeated reports of people with both Barrett's oesophagus and oesophageal cancer, the biggest series of reports being from the Mayo Clinic in the USA. There, Dr A. J. Cameron and colleagues found that 18 out of 122 people (15 per cent) with Barrett's oesophagus developed oesophageal cancer.

Although this sounds very high, when they followed up the

remaining 104 patients, only 2 more of them developed cancer – a 2 per cent rate. This is difficult to explain. In another series by S. J. Spechler and colleagues, only 2 out of 105 patients with Barrett's oesophagus developed oesophageal cancer over the next three years. Both were heavy smokers and drinkers who refused to stop their habits. Taking the two series together, the oesophageal cancer rate was still 40 times that expected of people without any known oesophageal disease, but the risk remained small for each individual.

The risk is even lower when it is considered that, of the patients with Barrett's oesophagus in these studies, 85 per cent were cigarette smokers and 76 per cent were 'addicted to alcohol'. As these two habits are known to raise the risk of oesophageal cancer, and may be instrumental in causing Barrett's oesophagus in the first place, it is difficult to calculate the risk, if there is any, of cancer if you have Barrett's oesophagus, do not smoke and only drink a little. What the reports do make very clear is that if you have a Barrett's oesophagus and you are a smoker and heavy drinker, you must stop.

Achalasia

Other conditions of the oesophagus that do not directly involve reflux, but may cause similar symptoms, include disorders of control of the swallowing muscles. Principal among these conditions is 'achalasia'. In achalasia, the oesophagus goes into 'spasm'. It's easiest to imagine as a form of cramp that affects the muscles of a segment of the oesophagus. People with achalasia have difficulty in swallowing, and this usually starts in childhood. At first they find it easier to swallow liquids than solids, but after a while most foods and drinks seem to 'stick' in the chest. If this state is allowed to continue, the oesophagus fills with food, like a balloon, and it suddenly empties upwards into the mouth.

That is bad enough, but if it occurs when you are sleeping you can breathe in the food and choke. Sufferers from achalasia may develop repeated chest infections, much like GORD sufferers, from repeated inhalation of food. In the early stages of achalasia, barium swallow X-rays show a bulging lower oesophagus above a short narrowed segment that does not open. Later, the bulge becomes much bigger as the oesophagus becomes a large soft bag of undigested food.

Achalasia is thought to be due to failure of the peristaltic wave to pass through the affected segment of the oesophagus, which remains narrow and underdeveloped. The fault lies either in the muscles themselves or in the nerves that co-ordinate their contraction and relaxation.

In the early stages of achalasia, the narrowed region can be stretched successfully by an instrument called a bougie or a water-filled dilator. If that isn't possible, and in the later stages of achalasia it usually isn't, then the patient needs surgery to re-fashion the oesophagus just above the cardia, and the cardia itself, to allow food to pass from the oesophagus into the stomach. The operation itself is called 'anterior myotomy' or the 'modified Heller' operation. It is usually highly successful in curing the achalasia, and the grateful patient is delighted to be able to swallow normally for the first time in his or her life.

Unfortunately, one of the drawbacks of any form of surgery for achalasia can be the beginning of GORD. The new cardia may allow so much room for passage of food down from the oesophagus into the stomach that there is also room for reflux in the opposite direction. So previous surgery for achalasia is a recognized cause of GORD. Most people who do develop it still prefer GORD to their previous discomfort: it is more easily managed and less of a disturbance to their lives.

Diffuse spasm

GORD may also be initiated by 'diffuse oesophageal spasm' and 'nutcracker oesophagus'. In diffuse spasm the peristaltic wave is normal through the whole oesophagus – this differentiates it from achalasia. However, from time to time there is an extra contraction in which the whole oesophagus goes into cramp. The muscles along its whole length contract at the same time, and stay in this cramp for several minutes before relaxing. The cramp causes a deep-seated pain in the centre of the chest that is often mistaken for angina or even a heart attack.

Nutcracker oesophagus

In nutcracker oesophagus, peristalsis, which is not normally an activity of which we are conscious, becomes much more powerful and lasts much longer than usual. It is so strong that it feels as if the cramping muscles could crack a nut between them – hence the name. X-rays taken at the time of the pain show very intense waves of contractions of the oesophageal muscles.

Both diffuse spasm and nutcracker oesophagus can be very

difficult to treat. Drugs to relieve spasm make little difference, and most sufferers from either condition need a regular insertion of a bougie (a ball-shaped dilator) into the oesophagus, or even surgery to cut the muscle fibres, to relieve their symptoms.

It now seems certain that many cases of diffuse spasms and nutcracker oesophagus are reactions to small amounts of acid passing by reflux up from the stomach into the lower oesophagus. Patients with these symptoms possess oesophageal mucosa that is extremely sensitive to acid, and the muscles surrounding it respond accordingly with cramp or exaggerated peristalsis. They are now treated with proton pump inhibitors that abolish the acid-producing property of the stomach.

Corkscrew oesophagus

A curious footnote to oesophageal disorders is 'corkscrew' oesophagus, a condition in which the oesophagus twists on itself, giving the appearance on X-ray of a corkscrew. This arises from a series of unco-ordinated contractions of oesophageal segments that do not help to propel the food downwards. Corkscrew oesophagus is sometimes linked, like nutcracker and diffuse spasms, to symptoms of GORD, but most of the time it causes no symptoms and is simply an odd X-ray finding of no significance.

Hiatus hernia

About 30 per cent of all people with GORD have a hiatus hernia that is partly responsible for their symptoms. In a hiatus hernia the cardia is lost, the angle between the lower oesophagus and the upper stomach straightens, and the sphincter no longer works. The positive pressure that keeps the lower oesophagus flat when there is no food above it has gone, so that it opens up enough to allow back-flow of the stomach's digestive juices. It is small wonder therefore that hiatus hernia leads to GORD, like night following day. It is important, therefore, that a hiatus hernia shouldn't be missed. However, even if it is repaired surgically, the operation doesn't necessarily cure all the symptoms. There may be residual problems with the sphincter that allow some to continue. Why this happens, and what should be done about it, is described in the chapter devoted to hiatus hernia.

First, however, it is important to understand why doctors don't seem to bother about investigating a case further if they think they have made the correct diagnosis from your collection of symptoms alone. That is the subject of the next chapter.

4

Treat or test? The crucial question

How best to treat GORD? Professors John Dent of the Royal
Adelaide Hospital, South Australia, Roger Jones, of Guy's, King's
and St Thomas's School of Medicine, London, Peter Kahrilas of the
Northwestern University Medical School, Chicago, and Nicholas
Tadley of the University of Sydney, combined to review the best
way to manage GORD in general practice.[4] They are distinguished
doctors whose deliberations were keenly read by doctors in hospital
and general practice as the definitive way forward for GORD in the
twenty-first century. Today, what they wrote is enshrined in the
guidance for good practice for all doctors in the UK. I have tried in
this chapter to put their advice to doctors into lay language. If you
have GORD, then this is the most important chapter for you to take
to heart. It explains why your doctor might not send you for tests –
and also why some people need tests and further investigations.

To begin with, in the usual style of medical reports in modern
journals, they made six key summary points that are worth repeating
here:

1 Careful analysis of symptoms and history is key to a diagnosis of
  GORD.
2 Diagnosis based on symptoms alone can be aided by a trial of
  treatment.
3 Clear endoscopic abnormalities are found in less than half of
  patients.
4 Treatment should start with the most effective therapy – a proton
  pump inhibitor.
5 Most patients will require long-term management, for which the
  guiding principle is to reduce to the least costly treatment that is
  effective in controlling symptoms.
6 Anti-reflux surgery may be as effective as long-term proton pump
  inhibitors, but is less predictable.

They then justified their conclusions by asking and answering a
series of questions. The two most important of them, for me, were:

- How reliable is diagnosis based on symptoms, and what can be done to aid it?
- When should a GP refer patients with the symptoms of GORD for further tests?

They made clear that GORD is completely different from other forms of dyspepsia, such as stomach and duodenal ulcers. The main symptoms of these 'peptic' ulcers are pain or discomfort in the upper abdomen, without heartburn. They based their diagnosis of GORD on the occurrence of heartburn on two or more days a week, although if it occurs less often, that still does not absolutely preclude it. They write that 'when heartburn is carefully defined it is unlikely to be due to anything other than gastro-oesophageal reflux disease. Three-quarters of patients in whom heartburn is the main or sole symptom have GORD.'[5] It is important that both doctor and patient understand exactly what heartburn is. Professor Dent and his colleagues found in their research that its description as 'a burning feeling rising from the stomach or lower chest up towards the neck' identified more patients with GORD than the simple use of the word 'heartburn'.

They justified their conclusion that most people with GORD as diagnosed from their symptoms alone do not need further tests on the basis of the finding that fewer than half of all patients with its symptoms have any abnormality on endoscopy. The use of endoscopy is only useful, therefore, in a minority.

So who are the minority for whom investigations such as endoscopy are essential? Professor Dent's team wrote that it is useful 'in some patients' to clarify diagnosis, assess severity of the disease, to recognize its complications and to define the best treatments, but they wrote that 'no consensus exists on its [i.e. endoscopy's] precise role or on whom, or when it is best performed'. They added that 'the use of endoscopy depends on local costs, accessibility and timing relative to treatment'.

How things have moved on since then! These days, all GPs in the UK are sent guidelines on how to manage people presenting with the symptoms of GORD, and they are strongly encouraged to act upon them.

The guidelines state:

- In patients under 55 years old with classical symptoms of

'heartburn', the history is sufficiently typical to permit a trial of therapy without the need for diagnostic tests.

- Always investigate if the patient is older than 55 with new symptoms . . .
- . . . or if a person of any age has 'alarm' symptoms such as weight loss; vomiting, bleeding or anaemia; dysphagia (difficulty in swallowing); persistent severe pain; an abdominal mass, or if changing the lifestyle does not help.

Every person with symptoms of GORD should have a simple blood test to rule out anaemia. If there is no anaemia, then the general rule, if the symptoms are not too severe, is for the patient to try a course of anti-reflux treatment (see Chapter 5). Only in exceptional cases does the doctor proceed to order further tests, the main one of which is endoscopy. We are moving away from other tests such as X-rays and measurements of pressures and acid levels inside the oesophagus, as they do not contribute much more than a good history to the assessment and diagnosis or, for that matter, the decision on the type of treatment.

Doctors will only send for further testing patients whom they see as perhaps needing extra attention, either because their symptoms are exceptionally severe or because they indicate some complication that needs specialist advice. They are covered in a later chapter.

Two 'scoring systems' that measure the severity of oesophagitis due to reflux disease have been popular with many doctors for some years (see Table 1). They serve as a guide on who should be referred to a specialist, and who can probably be treated simply on the basis of their symptoms alone.

One grades the three main symptoms of heartburn, regurgitation and swallowing difficulty in a four-point scale from none to severe. The other looks at frequency, duration and severity of each symptom in more detail. With either scale, the higher the eventual score, the more need there is for more effective treatment. Nowadays, that usually means a higher dose of a proton pump inhibitor, for which you should see the next chapter.

Table 1 Scoring systems for oesophagitis

The DeMeester scale:

Symptom	Grade	Description
Heartburn		
None	0	No heartburn
Mild	1	Occasional episodes
Moderate	2	Reason for visit to doctor
Severe	3	Enough to interfere with daily life
Regurgitation		
None	0	No regurgitation
Mild	1	Occasional episodes
Moderate	2	Predictable on moving position or straining
Severe	3	Associated with night-time cough or pneumonia
Swallowing difficulty (dysphagia)		
None	0	No dysphagia
Mild	1	Occasional episodes
Moderate	2	Needs a drink to clear it
Severe	3	At least one episode of obstruction needing medical treatment

The Jamieson and Duranceau scale:

	One point	Two points	Three points	Four points
Frequency	Under once a month	More than once a month but less than weekly	More than once a week, but not daily	Every day
Duration	Less than 6 months	More than 6 months, less than 24 months	More than 24 months, less than 60 months	More than 60 months
Severity	Nuisance value only	Spoils enjoyment of life	Interferes with normal living	Worst possible symptoms

(*Note*: This scale is used for each symptom in turn – heartburn, dysphagia, chest pain, regurgitation, and breathing problems.)

There is controversy over what the next step should be for anyone who scores high on these scales. Should he or she be sent for a barium swallow, or go straight for an endoscopy? What is the place for acid and pressure measurements – tests that were often used until recently?

In the barium X-ray, the patient swallows while the radiologist watches the moving film. The changing shape of the lump of barium passing down the oesophagus can show up problems of mobility, such as achalasia and spasm. It can show reflux spilling upwards through the cardia, and can even indicate inflammation in the lower oesophagus. However, on its own it is not always reliable as an indicator of reflux disease. Studies have failed to connect reflux with oesophagitis: some patients with reflux have no oesophagitis, and others with no reflux are found on endoscopy to have severe oesophagitis. Techniques involving patients having to change position from one side to another and from horizontal to vertical are used to see whether the cardia is opening properly. Sometimes food is given as well as the barium to try to stimulate reflux. How far reflux travels up the oesophagus during a barium X-ray may determine how you are treated.

Refined barium X-rays include a 'double-contrast' technique, which involves the patient swallowing some barium very quickly and then the oesophagus is distended with gas from a fizzy powder. In a variation on this technique, you are asked first to swallow a tablespoonful of alkaline solution, then about half a cup of barium, a tablespoon of an acid solution, and three drops of a 'bubble-breaker'. Double-contrast X-rays show the lining of the oesophagus in great detail, even highlighting small ulcers. The radiologist has a very clear picture of the extent of the reflux and how much damage it has done to the oesophagus.

So barium swallow X-rays are still of value. However, few patients are now subjected to the measurements of pressure or acid inside the oesophagus that I wrote about in detail when first writing about hiatus hernia in 1997 (*Coping Successfully with Your Hiatus Hernia*, Sheldon Press). These tests are now virtually restricted to volunteers in research programmes, and patients can be thankful that they are, because they were quite difficult to tolerate.

The UK 2005 guidelines advise that the main investigation is endoscopy, and Professor Dent and his colleagues list the indications for early endoscopy as follows:

- Alarm symptoms as above.
- When the diagnosis is in doubt, as with atypical symptoms.
- When the symptoms do not disappear with the initial treatment.
- As an assessment before surgery for hiatus hernia.
- To reassure patients when they are unable to accept verbal advice.

Professor Dent and his colleagues add that endoscopy may also be appropriate when people have had frequent, troublesome symptoms for a long time, in order to 'tailor' the drug treatment to the endoscopy findings, and to detect and manage Barrett's oesophagus (see the previous chapter).

Endoscopy

The flexible fibre-optic endoscope has made a huge contribution to our knowledge of medicine, and nowhere more so than for patients with GORD. It is a fully flexible tube inside of which is a bundle of glass fibres through which the operator can see very clearly what is going on inside the throat, oesophagus and stomach. It also allows instruments to be passed along its length so that biopsies (pieces of tissue) can be taken at specific points in the full view of the operator, for microscopic examination.

It is passed under local anaesthetic into the oesophagus. It may sound horrendous to have such a procedure without a general anaesthetic, but the sedative makes you so drowsy beforehand that you hardly feel the discomfort and will have very little memory of it afterwards.

Endoscopy gives its operator a magnified view of what is happening over the whole length of the oesophagus, the cardia and the stomach. It is used for diagnosis, to assess the severity and the extent of the oesophagitis, and to relate the site of the cardia to the level of the diaphragm. This point is seen as the Z-line, a sharp difference in appearance of the surface as the oesophageal lining becomes the stomach lining.

In 1997, in the book on hiatus hernia that I mentioned above, I wrote: 'the experts still disagree on how to assess the severity of oesophagitis. They have partly agreed on a classification which helps them to decide on how to proceed with treatment.'

In 2005, there is much more agreement on how to assess

oesophagitis. There are now two standard ways of grading oesophagitis by endoscopy appearance. The first, the Los Angeles classification system, depends entirely on the appearance of the oesophageal mucosa to the naked eye, grading it into one of four classes. The operator is asked to assess the length of breaks (small erosions, leading to larger ulcers, produced by inflammation) in the mucosa, and relates them to the 'folds' in the lining that are a normal feature of the oesophagus. An ulcer that extends more than the distance between the folds is looked on as more serious than a shorter one. The second system, the Savary-Miller classification, uses five grades that encompass what the operator sees plus the microscopic appearance on biopsy. The British guidelines recommend both, leaving it to local hospital staff doctors to decide which one to use. Our local hospital uses the Savary-Miller system, which seems to be more comprehensive. I give both here, for completeness, and to help you understand the grounds on which your treatment has been decided.

Endoscopy grading systems

Los Angeles classification

Grade of oesophagitis
(A) One or more mucosal breaks no longer than 5 mm, none of which extends between the tops of the mucosal folds.
(B) One or more mucosal breaks more than 5 mm long, none of which extends between the tops of the mucosal folds.
(C) Mucosal breaks that extend between the tops of two or more mucosal folds, but which involve less than 75 per cent of the oesophageal circumference.
(D) Mucosal breaks that involve at least 75 per cent of the oesophageal circumference.

Savary-Miller classification

Grade of oesophagitis
1 Single or multiple erosions on a single fold: erosions may be erythematous (red) or exudative (covered with fluid).
2 Multiple erosions affecting multiple folds: erosions may be confluent (joining together).
3 Multiple circumferential erosions (that extend around the oesophagus like a ring).

4 Ulcer, stenosis or oesophageal shortening.
5 Barrett's epithelium, in which the epithelium shows a change from the normal appearance (the microscopic diagnosis of the biopsy shows 'columnar epithelium') in the form of circular or non-circular ('islands' or 'tongues') extensions of erosions.

Either classification gives the specialist a guide to the treatment needed, which is explained in the next chapter.

The endoscopy will also help in diagnosing other causes of GORD symptoms. They include oesophagitis from swallowed corrosive substances, which, as mentioned in the previous chapter, includes painkilling drugs such as aspirin and NSAIDs, often prescribed for the chronic pain of, say, arthritis. Other diagnoses confirmed by endoscopy are infection, especially in people with immune diseases such as AIDS (who may get virus and fungal infections of the oesophagus that are not a risk for people with normal immune systems). Cancers, stomach ulcers, non-ulcer dyspepsia and oesophageal spasm (see the previous chapter) are also diagnosed from endoscopy.

5

Treating GORD – who and how?

The first priority the doctor has in treating GORD is to reassure you that you have every chance that the symptoms will ease and even disappear. You, though, have your part to play in your own treatment by changing your lifestyle, and your doctor will help by supporting you with effective drugs. Once treatment starts, you will also be reassured that you don't have an illness that is life-threatening. Many people with GORD are frightened that they may have cancer or heart disease: once your diagnosis has been made clear you can cast these worries aside and get on with your life, content in the knowledge that GORD can be beaten. Once you understand that, you are already treating yourself and the cure has started before you have swallowed your first pill.

The wrong lifestyle has played its part in most people with GORD, and changing to a healthier lifestyle is the first step towards cure for most of them. The guidelines on lifestyle for GORD include:

- Lose excess weight.
- Stop smoking.
- Reduce alcohol intake if it is above two standard drinks (of wine) a day.
- Raise the head of the bed at night and use plenty of pillows (to try to stay reasonably upright when asleep).
- Eat small meals often, rather than one large meal at any time.
- Avoid hot drinks.
- Avoid alcohol and food less than three hours before going to bed at night (to avoid a full stomach when lying horizontal).
- Avoid drugs that may affect the normal peristalsis of the oesophagus or the sphincter (nitrates, anticholinergics, tricyclic antidepressants).
- Avoid drugs that may damage the oesophageal mucosa (NSAIDs, potassium salts, bisphosphonates).

There are four points to make about this comprehensive list. The first is about losing weight.

49

Losing weight

If you can exercise easily without bringing on a cough or wheezing, do so. The best way is to find an exercise that you enjoy (cycling, swimming, brisk walking, ballroom dancing – it doesn't matter as long as you are likely to stick to it), and do it for at least half an hour, preferably an hour, on three or four days a week. It should be brisk enough to make you breathless, without causing you distress. If you can manage this regimen, you will find that you can lose a pound or two each week – and that amounts to 50 pounds a year! If this is combined with eating smaller amounts, it will ease your discomfort from an over-full stomach and decrease the pressure inside the abdomen that tends to push your stomach contents upwards.

The secret of losing weight by eating less is to eat *slowly*. Most fat people tend to wolf down their food, taking 15 minutes or less to polish off a large meal at home. If they could spread the time to more than half an hour, they would eat a lot less.

The reason for this is that once we feel hungry, it takes about half an hour for the feeling to die down, no matter how much we eat (within reason). If we eat our main meals around a table, having conversation with friends and family, eating slowly and waiting between courses, the feeling of satiety (fullness) starts in around half an hour, regardless of how much we have eaten (provided, of course, we have eaten something!). So if we eat slowly enough, we feel full before we have eaten a large amount, and we lose weight.

We in the UK seem to have abandoned this habit of eating around the family table, and we face a huge problem of obesity. The French eat as they have always done, taking their time and savouring every bite. Go to Paris and try to spot an obese adult – he or she is much more likely to be a tourist than a local. The French are far less affected by the obesity plague than we are.

Which foods?

The second point is that it doesn't really matter, within reason, what food you eat. People with digestive problems often ask which foods cause their symptoms and which are unlikely to do so. They are surprised to find that there are very few types of food that cause GORD symptoms. A minority of sufferers find that fried foods upset them: others find that tea or coffee or similar hot drinks do so.

Many more rue the glass of spirits that well-meaning friends have offered them. The rule about food is that if you find one that brings on heartburn or discomfort, then avoid it. Everyone is different. It is more important to eat a variety of foods that don't obviously induce the symptoms rather than to go on a restrictive diet. You will almost certainly find, as you change from big meals to small portions eaten slowly, that you return to eating foods that in the past you thought made you feel ill. This is why there is no chapter or section in this book dedicated to diets. They don't work in GORD, except in so far as you will find by trial and experience which foods suit you and which ones don't.

Sleeping position

The third point is about raising the head of the bed. Of course, it is meant to keep the upper body semi-upright, to avoid reflux passing horizontally from stomach to oesophagus. I've found in practice that all it does is to make people slide down the bed while they sleep so that they end up curled up, flat on the mattress. That is no advantage to them, and can result in a disturbed night. So I would add that if you are going to raise the bed head, do it by only 2 or 3 inches, and put a foot-plate at the bottom of the bed, so you can't slip downwards. To be frank, raising the bed doesn't often help: if you really have to keep upright overnight, you may well find that sleeping in an easy chair with a back and side arms is more effective. Once your lifestyle changes have started to improve your symptoms, you can then return to bed, using two or three pillows to keep your body at a reasonable angle from the horizontal.

Smoking

My fourth point is a very serious one – about smoking. Smoking has such a bad effect on GORD that I felt that it deserved a separate chapter to itself. If you smoke, the next chapter is a vital one for you. If you don't smoke, at least let relatives or friends who smoke read it, because the message to stop is just as much a general one as it is specifically aimed at GORD.

6

Why, if you smoke,
you absolutely *must* stop

According to the studies on GORD, more than 80 per cent of sufferers smoke, many of them heavily. That in itself makes a point – as fewer than 30 per cent of those in most developed countries now smoke, there must be a strong link between smoking and GORD.

Smoking is a stupid, suicidal habit for anyone, no matter how healthy. It is even worse, if that is possible, for people with GORD, because it irritates the already inflamed oesophagus and prevents it healing. It narrows the already compromised circulation to the affected area of oesophagus, something you absolutely can't afford to happen, as it increases the risk of a haemorrhage or a perforation from it. Worst of all, smoking increases the acid production in the stomach and damages the mucosal protective barrier of mucus. In every way, even smoking one or two cigarettes a day will reduce your chances of dealing successfully with GORD. So if you are a smoker, you *must* become a non-smoker before you put this book down.

How, exactly, does being a smoker harm you? Tobacco smoke contains carbon monoxide and nicotine. The first poisons the red blood cells, so that they cannot pick up and distribute much-needed oxygen to the organs and tissues, including the heart muscle. Carbon monoxide-affected red cells (in the 20-a-day smoker, nearly 20 per cent of red cells are carrying carbon monoxide instead of oxygen) are also stiffer than normal, so that they can't bend and flex through the smallest blood vessels. The gas also directly poisons the heart muscle, so that it cannot contract properly and efficiently, thereby delivering a 'double whammy' of damage to it.

Nicotine causes small arteries to narrow, so that the blood flow through them slows. It raises blood cholesterol levels, thickening the blood and promoting degeneration in artery walls. Both nicotine and carbon monoxide encourage the blood to clot, multiplying the risks of coronary thrombosis and stroke.

Add to all this the tars that smoke leaves in the lungs, which further reduce the ability of red cells to pick up oxygen, and the scars and damage to the lungs that always in the end produce chronic bronchitis and sometimes induces cancer, and you have a formula for disaster.

Smoking – the facts

Here are the bald facts about smoking. If what you have already read above about smoking and GORD, and about the malign effects of smoking on your general health, have not convinced you to stop, then you may as well give up reading this book, because there is no point in being 'health conscious' if you continue to indulge in tobacco. Its ill effects will counterbalance any good that your doctors can do for you.

- Smoking causes more deaths from heart attacks than from lung cancer and bronchitis.
- People who smoke have two or three times the risk of a fatal heart attack than non-smokers. The risk increases with the rising number of cigarettes smoked.
- Men under 45 who smoke 25 or more cigarettes a day have a 10 to 15 times greater chance of death from a heart attack than male non-smokers of the same age.
- About 40 per cent of all heavy smokers die before they reach 65. Of those who reach that age, many are disabled by bronchitis, angina, heart failure and leg amputations, all because they smoked. Only 10 per cent of smokers survive in reasonable health to the age of 75. Most non-smokers reach 75 in good health.
- In Britain, 40 per cent of all cancer deaths are from lung cancer, which is very rare in non-smokers. Of 441 British male doctors who died from lung cancer, only 7 had never smoked. Only 1 non-smoker in 60 develops lung cancer: the figure for heavy smokers is 1 in 6!
- Other cancers more common in smokers than in non-smokers include tongue, throat, larynx, pancreatic, kidney, bladder and cervix cancers.

The very fact that you are reading this book means that you are taking an intelligent interest in your health. So, after reading so far, it should be common sense to you not to smoke. Yet it is very difficult to stop, and many people who need an excuse for not stopping put up spurious arguments for their stance. Here are ones that every doctor is tired of hearing, and my replies to them:

- *My father/grandfather smoked 20 a day and lived till he was 75.* Everyone knows someone like that, but they conveniently forget the many others they have known who died long before their time. The chances are that you will be one of those, rather than one of the lucky few.
- *People who don't smoke also have heart attacks.* True. There are other causes of heart attacks, but 70 per cent of all people under 65 admitted to coronary care with heart attacks are smokers, as are 91 per cent of people with angina considered for coronary bypass surgery.
- *I believe in moderation in all things, and I only smoke moderately.* That's rubbish. We don't accept moderation in mugging, or dangerous driving, or exposure to asbestos (which incidentally causes far fewer deaths from lung cancer than smoking). Younger men who are only moderate smokers have a much higher risk of having a heart attack than non-smoking men of the same age. The figures are even worse for women.
- *I can cut down on cigarettes, but I can't stop.* It won't do you much good if you do. People who cut down usually inhale more from each cigarette and leave a smaller butt, so that they end up with the same blood levels of nicotine and carbon monoxide. You must stop completely.
- *I'm just as likely to be run over in the road as to die from my smoking.* In the UK, about 15 people die on the roads each day. This contrasts with 100 deaths a day from lung cancer, 100 from chronic bronchitis, and 100 from heart attacks, almost all of which are due to smoking. Of every 1,000 young men who smoke, on average 1 will be murdered, 6 will die on the roads, and 250 will die from their smoking habit.
- *I have to die from something.* In my experience this is always said by someone in good health. They no longer say it after their heart attack or stroke, or after they have coughed up blood.
- *I don't want to be old, anyway.* We define 'old' differently as we grow older. Most of us would like to live a long time, without the inconvenience of being old. If we take care of ourselves on the way to becoming old we have at least laid the foundations for enjoying our old age.

- *I'd rather die of a heart attack than something else.* Most of us would like a fast, sudden death, but many heart attack victims leave a grieving partner in their early fifties to face 30 years of loneliness. Is that really what you want?
- *Stress, not smoking, is the main cause of heart attacks.* Not true. Stress is very difficult to measure and it is very hard to relate it to heart attack rates. In any case, you have to cope with stress, whether you smoke or not. Smoking is an extra burden that can never help, and it does not relieve stress. It isn't burning the candle at both ends that does the harm, but burning the cigarette at one end.
- *I'll stop when I start to feel ill.* That would be fine if the first sign of illness were not a full-blown heart attack from which more than a third die in the first four hours. It's too late to stop then.
- *I'll put on weight if I stop smoking.* You probably will, because your appetite will return and you will be able to taste food again. But if you have read the section in this book about changing your eating habits to control your weight better, than you will lose any extra weight anyway. In any case, the benefits of stopping smoking far outweigh the few extra pounds you may put on.
- *I enjoy smoking and don't want to give it up.* Is that really true? Is that not just an excuse because you can't stop? Ask yourself what your real pleasure is in smoking, and try to be honest with the answer.
- *Cigarettes settle my nerves. If I stopped, I'd have to take a tranquillizer.* Smoking is a prop, like a baby's dummy, but it solves nothing. It doesn't remove any causes of stress, and only makes things worse because it is another promoter of bad health. And when you start to have symptoms, like the regular morning cough, it only makes you worry more. It will also make it more difficult for you to control your weight.
- *I'll change to a pipe or cigar – they are safer.* Lifelong pipe and cigar smokers are less prone than cigarette smokers to heart attacks, but have five times the risk of lung cancer, and ten times the risk of chronic bronchitis, than non-smokers. Cigarette smokers who switch to pipes or cigars continue to be at high risk of a heart attack, probably because they inhale.
- *I've been smoking now for 30 years – it's too late to stop now.* It's not too late, whenever you stop. The risk of sudden death from a first heart attack falls away very quickly after stopping, even after

a lifetime of smoking. If you stop after surviving a heart attack, then you halve the risk of a second one. It takes longer to reduce your risk of lung cancer, but it falls by 80 per cent over the next 15 years, no matter how long you have been a smoker.

- *I wish I could stop. I've tried everything, but nothing has worked.* Stopping smoking isn't easy unless you really want to do it. You have to make the effort yourself, rather than think that someone else can do it for you. So you must be motivated. If the next few pages do not motivate you, then nothing will.

Stopping smoking

You yourself must find the right reason to stop smoking. For someone with GORD, it should surely include the fact that you may feel much better and have far fewer symptoms if you stop, and will be giving yourself a much better chance of remaining healthy for much longer. But there are plenty of other reasons to stop smoking.

If you are a young adult or teenager, who sees middle age and sickness as remote possibilities, and smoking as exciting and dangerous, the best attacks on smoking are the way it makes you look and smell. You can also add the environmental pollution of cigarette ends and the way big business exploits Third World nations, keeping their populations in poverty while they make huge profits by putting land that should be growing food under tobacco cultivation. Pakistan uses 120,000 acres, and Brazil half a million acres of their richest agricultural land, to grow tobacco. And as the multinationals are now promoting their product very heavily to the developing world, no teenager who smokes can claim to be really concerned about the health of the Third World. Is this as persuasive an argument for you to stop (or not to start) as any about health or looks?

If you are a more mature woman, looks may be the key. Smoking ages you prematurely, causing wrinkles and giving a pale, pasty complexion. If you smoke you will probably experience the menopause at an earlier age than normal, even in your mid-thirties, which can destroy your plans to have your family after a career.

For men and older women, the prime motivation is better health. The statistics for men and women in their sixties who smoke are frightening. More than a third of men who smoke fail to reach pension age.

How to stop

Let us assume you are now fully motivated. How do you stop? It is easy. You become a non-smoker, as if you have never smoked. You throw away all your cigarettes, and decide never to buy or accept another one. Announce the fact to all your friends, who will usually support you, and that's that. Most people find that they don't have true withdrawal symptoms, provided they are happy to stop. A few become agitated, irritable, nervous and can't sleep at night. But people who have had to stop for medical reasons – say, because they have been admitted to coronary care – hardly ever have withdrawal symptoms.

That strongly suggests that the withdrawal problems are psychological, rather than physical. If you can last a week or two without a smoke, you will probably never light up again. The desire to smoke will disappear as the levels of carbon monoxide, nicotine and tarry chemicals in your lungs, blood, brain and other organs gradually subside.

If you must stop gradually, plan ahead. Keep a diary of the cigarettes you will have, leaving out one or two each succeeding day, and stick to it. Carry nicotine chewing gum or get a patch if you must, but remember that the nicotine is still harmful. Don't look on it as a long-term alternative to smoking. If you are having real difficulty stopping, ask your doctor for a prescription of Zyban. You may be offered a two-month course of the drug. It helps, but is by no means infallible.

If you do use aids to stop (other methods include acupuncture and hypnosis), remember they have no magical properties. They are a crutch to lean on while you make the determined effort to stop altogether. They cannot help if your will to stop is weak.

Recognize, too, that stopping smoking is not an end in itself. It is only part of your new way of life, one that includes your new way of eating and exercise, and your new attitude to your future health. And you owe it not only to yourself but also to your partner, family and friends, because it will help to give them a healthier you for, hopefully, years to come. You are not on your own. More than a million Britons have stopped smoking each year for the last 15 years. Only one in three adults now smokes (fewer than one in 20 doctors). By stopping you are joining the sensible majority.

7

The medical treatment of GORD

Happily, drugs do work in GORD. There are five groups of drugs, listed in order of efficacy by the GP guidelines and by Professor Dent and his team. Table 2 is adapted from the guidelines.

Table 2 Drug treatments for GORD
(in ascending order of effectiveness and cost)

1 Antacids and alginates.
2 H^2 receptor antagonists (such as ranitidine and cimetidine).
3 'As needed' doses of proton pump inhibitors (such as omeprazole and lansoprazole).
4 Maintenance low-dose proton pump inhibitors.
5 Healing high-dose proton pump inhibitors.

Antacids and alginates

Antacids describe themselves. They are alkaline medicines designed to neutralize the acid produced by the stomach. Alginates are derived from seaweed (agar) and are designed to release a gel into the lower oesophagus that will protect the surface from acid attack, or act as a 'raft' that floats on the top of the stomach contents and prevent the upward flow into the oesophagus. Both types of treatment, especially if given together, are effective for mild to moderate GORD.

Antacids are usually aluminium or magnesium compounds. They range in convenience and cost – the cheaper preparations tending to be less palatable than, but just as effective as, the dearer ones. They can all be bought from pharmacies to save you having to wait for a prescription.

The basic antacids are aluminium hydroxide and magnesium carbonate or trisilicate. Pharmacies have dozens of formulations of them to suit your taste and preference. Co-magaldrox is a mixture of aluminium and magnesium hydroxides, marketed as Maalox or Mucogel. Aluminium and magnesium compounds are poorly soluble in water, and act for a long time if they remain in the stomach. The main difference between them is that aluminium-containing antacids tend to constipate and magnesium compounds tend to loosen the motions, so combining them, in theory, minimizes these effects on the bowel.

If you need a longer action, you can choose a combination of an antacid with an alginate. The sticky alkaline barrier that they form on the top of the stomach contents combines neutralization of the acid with the raft principle mentioned above. Among alginate-containing products are Algicon, Gastrocote, Gaviscon, Peptac, Rennie Duo and Topal. There are many more.

An alternative to alginate is a silicone, such as simeticone (dimeticone). This is a 'de-foaming' agent that is thought to make it easier to belch, reduce bloating, and allow faster passage of food and digestive juices through the stomach, reducing reflux as it does so. It is particularly useful in easing hiccups. Antacid-simeticone preparations include Altacite Plus, Asilone and Maalox Plus. Again, there are many others.

All antacid-alginate or antacid-simeticone combinations are popular over-the-counter drugs, so they must work for many people. If you find one that suits you, you may as well stick to it. However, if you have to take one every day, you need to step up your treatment into the acid-suppressant drugs, the H^2 receptor antagonists or the proton pump inhibitors.

H^2 receptor antagonists

Acid-suppressant drugs act on the acid-producing mechanisms within the stomach wall, so that, in the case of H^2 receptor antagonists, they greatly reduce the amount of acid inside the stomach. This is more effective in easing symptoms for most people with moderate to severe oesophagitis than antacid combinations.

Cimetidine (Tagamet) was the first of this group of drugs. It revolutionized the treatment of gastric and duodenal ulcers, but it was marginally less successful when tried against reflux oesophagitis. Patients taking it in the early trials found that their symptoms were much less, but endoscopy appearances showed that they still had a moderate degree of inflammation in the oesophagus. The early doses were possibly too low, and many people with reflux have to take double the original dose of 400 mg to keep their symptoms at bay.

Ranitidine (Zantac) was the second H^2 antagonist. It is similar in effect to cimetidine, and the usual dose is 300 mg each evening. The dose can be raised up to as much as 1500 mg daily for added benefit, although most doctors would prefer not to go so high, and use another treatment, probably a proton pump inhibitor, instead.

Newer H^2 antagonists include famotidine (Pepcid) and nizatidine (Axid). They are similar in action to cimetidine and ranitidine, with little to choose between them.

All drugs may produce side-effects, and acid-suppressant drugs are no exception. H^2 receptor antagonists should be used with caution in people with liver or kidney problems or who are pregnant or breast feeding. They may 'mask' the symptoms of stomach cancer, so if you have one or more of the 'alarm' symptoms described in Chapter 4, your specialist will rule out stomach cancer before prescribing one. Side-effects of this group of drugs are relatively rare, but they include diarrhoea, headache, dizziness, rash and tiredness. Much rarer are effects on the heart rhythm, on the bone marrow and occasional reports of enlarged breasts in men (gynaecomastia) and impotence. Cimetidine has a disadvantage compared with other drugs in this group, in that it interacts with drugs that use the same type of mechanism in the liver for their breakdown. So it cannot be taken alongside warfarin (an anti-clotting drug), phenytoin (for epilepsy) or theophylline (for asthma). The other drugs in this group may be taken instead.

Proton pump inhibitors

Proton pump inhibitors (PPIs) act on the acid-producing mechanism at an earlier stage in the process than H^2 antagonists, so that they completely eradicate acid, rather than reduce it, from the stomach contents. The first PPI was omeprazole (Losec). It has since been joined by esomeprazole (Nexium), lansoprazole (Zoton), pantoprazole (Protium) and rabeprazole (Pariet).

As with the H^2 antagonists, PPIs are so efficient in removing symptoms in reflux disease, even when it is severe, that they can 'mask' a stomach cancer. When a person shows 'alarm features' (see Chapter 4) the specialist team must rule out a stomach or oesophageal cancer before prescribing them. Side-effects of PPIs are similar to those of the H^2 antagonists. The patient leaflet for PPIs list all the side-effects that have been reported: they look horrendous, but it must be remembered that they are all very rare. Most people find them easy to tolerate and that they have no side-effects. However, it is important to read the leaflet, so that if a problem does arise, you can tell what it is, and deal with it accordingly.

Which drug?

With all these drugs to choose from, how do doctors decide which is the right one for you? This is where the 'guidelines' from NICE (the National Institute for Clinical Excellence) are so helpful.

NICE recommends either a 'step up' or a 'step down' approach, depending on the severity of the illness. If you look again at Table 2 earlier in this chapter, you will see that it has five levels, starting with the mildest treatment (antacids/alginates) through H^2 antagonists, to rising doses of PPIs. For example, if endoscopy has shown that you have ulcers in your oesophagus or Barrett's oesophagus, you will start on the highest 'healing' dose of a PPI – level 5. The dose can eventually be cut down once the symptoms have improved, to a level that continues to keep you symptom-free. On the other hand, if you have mild symptoms and no need for endoscopy, you may be started on level 1, with an antacid-alginate combination and advised on lifestyle. If this does not work, your doctor may add an H^2 antagonist – level 2. Depending on your progress after that, you will pass up or down the scale. All patients should have their own 'treatment plan' that guides them on how to manage their own symptoms, and this can often be stopped when their oesophagus eventually heals and the symptoms disappear.

However, the fact that you are able to stop the treatment doesn't mean that you can now stop going to your doctor. As Professor Dent's team wrote in their review:

> Most people with gastro-oesophageal reflux disease require long term management. The guiding principle for long term management is to step down to the treatment that is least costly but still effective in controlling symptoms. Finding the right level of management may take time in some patients. Patients returning with a relapse after a trial without treatment should be restarted on the initially successful therapy and then have treatment stepped down as appropriate. For patients who require only intermittent short courses of antisecretory (acid-lowering) therapy, it may be more effective to give a proton pump inhibitor at full dose than to titrate treatment up from either half dose of PPI or a standard dose of H^2 receptor antagonist.

Professor Dent is also against repeated endoscopy. He states that by optimizing the treatment in these 'steps', endoscopy is kept to a minimum. If a particular treatment successfully controls a patient's symptoms, the doctor can be assured that the oesophagitis has healed, and there is no need for further endoscopies. Even when the patient needs to continue on long-term PPIs because of severe oesophagitis (Los Angeles stages (C) and (D)), repeat endoscopy is not always needed, as it is safe to assume that if the symptoms are absent, the oesophagitis has healed. On the other hand, patients in these categories must have repeat endoscopies if they still have symptoms despite standard daily doses of PPIs.

The groups of patients who must be kept on continuous treatment include:

- Patients with ulcers in the oesophagus that have been induced by an NSAID and who have no choice but to continue with it because they have chronic pain (such as from arthritis). They should remain on maintenance doses of PPIs (level 4).
- Patients with severe GORD, such as Barrett's oesophagus or an endoscopy-proven ulcer, should also remain on maintenance doses of a PPI (level 4).
- Patients whose very severe reflux disease has been complicated in the past by stricture, ulcers and haemorrhage should be left on full doses of PPIs (level 5).

'Prokinetic' drugs, designed to speed up the passage of food from stomach to duodenum, such as metoclopramide (Maxolon, Gastro-bid) can be added, if needed, to help prevent bloating.

If things get worse

Most people, once they start their treatment for GORD, do very well. They remain symptom-free and can live normal lives. However, they should remain on their doctor's follow-up list, even if they have been able to stop their medicines. That's because, with a history of GORD, you are at slightly higher risk than the rest of the population of complications, the most serious of which is oesophageal cancer. You should be aware of the warning signs that you need to seek urgent help.

The United Kingdom Department of Health has issued guidelines for doctors on who, and what symptoms, should be referred to a specialist urgently because of suspected upper gastro-intestinal cancer. They include:

- Dysphagia – food sticking on swallowing, at any age.
- Dyspepsia (indigestion) at any age, combined with one or more of the following 'alarm' symptoms: weight loss, proven anaemia (from a blood count), or vomiting.
- Dyspepsia in a patient aged 55* or over with at least one of the following 'high-risk' features: onset of the dyspepsia less than a year before, continuous symptoms since it started.
- Dyspepsia combined with at least one of the following known 'risk factors': a family history of oesophageal or stomach cancer in more than two close relatives, Barrett's oesophagus, pernicious anaemia (a condition in which the stomach cannot produce acid), ulcer surgery more than 20 years before, and known changes in the lining of the stomach or oesophagus (a condition called dysplasia or atrophic gastritis).
- Jaundice.
- A mass in the upper abdomen.

*55 years is the maximum age at which health care authorities set the threshold for investigation. Many local cancer networks set a lower threshold of the age of 50, or even 45.

If you recognize yourself to be in one of these categories, or do so in the future, you must immediately contact your doctor. You will be offered an endoscopy within two weeks of doing so, and it will probably be arranged even sooner.

Professor Dent and his colleagues end their report with their thoughts on surgery for GORD. Surgery to correct reflux, they write, 'is an attractive option for some patients as it can eliminate the need for life-long drug treatment'. So it isn't just reserved for patients in whom drug treatment has failed. A review comparing the results, over five years, of long-term drug treatment and corrective surgery has reported that the two are equally effective in producing a cure.[6] Whether you opt for surgery or long-term drug treatment is as much up to your own preference as to the doctor's. The statistics suggest that long-term proton pump therapy is marginally safer than surgery, which has a small mortality rate of around 2 per 1,000 operations, so one of the questions about surgery that you must be able to answer for yourself is: 'Do I think the small extra risk is worth it?' You can only answer that question for yourself. If you opt for surgery to relieve your GORD, you must understand all the risks that are relevant to you beforehand, and sign a paper of consent to the operation in the full knowledge of those risks. This is what the next chapter is about.

8

Surgery for GORD

Back in 1991, Dr B. Dallemagne and his colleagues published the first report of a series of operations designed to cure GORD.[7] It started a new era for people with GORD whose symptoms were not well controlled by medicines. The aim of the surgery is to re-establish the tone in the gastro-oesophageal sphincter by wrapping the fundus of the stomach around the part of the lower oesophagus that is below the diaphragm – the last 5 centimetres. The 'wrap' is then 'anchored' below the diaphragm, inside the abdomen with three non-absorbable stitches. The crura are also stitched securely around the hiatus, making sure that the oesophagus is neatly surrounded by muscle that will prevent reflux.

The original operation is called the 'Nissen fundoplication' – it is named after the surgeon who invented it. Other surgeons have opted for variations: they are the Toupet and Hill operations. If you are opting for surgery, your surgeon will let you know which his team favours.

The operation is performed either as open surgery (in which case there is a long wound) or by laparoscopy (using a fibre-optic tube through which the surgeon can manipulate the instruments). Laparoscopy in the hands of a skilled surgeon gives similar results to open surgery, but it leaves you more comfortable afterwards, with less pain and a shorter stay in hospital.

In January 2000, 11 professors and leading surgeons throughout the Netherlands reported, in the *Lancet*, their findings on behalf of the Netherlands Antireflux Surgery Study Group.[8] They chose patients with symptoms of GORD who had not improved well enough on at least 40 mg of omeprazole daily, with persisting oesophagus and proven acid exposure in the lower part of the oesophagus. The patients were first asked to double or triple their daily omeprazole dose, and most responded to this. If the symptoms returned when the dose was lowered again to 40 mg daily, they were asked if they wanted surgery. The surgeons also included a group of patients who were unwilling to take drugs for life to suppress their symptoms. To be considered for surgery, the patients had to be between 18 and 65 years old.

It is important to understand here that the operation is not performed just in people with proven hiatus hernia. The patients were chosen on the basis of their symptoms – heartburn and regurgitation – and on their severity. On average, they had had GORD symptoms for around four years. Because this was a trial comparing laparoscopic with open surgery, they had investigations that would not normally be done routinely for the average GORD patient. For example, pressures were measured in the oesophagus and across the sphincter, peristalsis was recorded, and the amount of acid washing back up the oesophagus was measured. On endoscopy, more than half of them had no oesophagitis – proof, if it were needed, that the symptoms of GORD do not necessarily reflect the severity of the damage to the oesophagus.

Fewer than half of the patients, too, had evidence of hiatus hernia. Fundoplication is just as effective, it appears, in people who simply have a weak gastro-oesophageal sphincter as in those with a hiatus hernia. More than two-thirds of the patients in each group showed serious acid reflux into the oesophagus – in the laparoscopy group of 57 patients, 12.4 per cent of the oesophageal surface had been exposed to acid. The corresponding figure before surgery for the 46 patients in the open surgery group was 11.6 per cent. Three months after the surgery, the acid reflux was measured again. It had dropped to 1.8 and 1.6 per cent respectively, to about a tenth of the previous measurements.

These are excellent results for both operations. The surgeons estimated that reflux control had been achieved in 96.5 per cent of the laparoscopy group and 98 per cent of the open surgery group, not a significant difference between the two types of operation, and a very high degree of success.

Yet there was a problem. Seven patients allocated to laparoscopy, but none of the patients given open surgery, developed dysphagia afterwards. They had replaced their heartburn with difficulty in swallowing. The surgeons had to score the success rate for laparoscopy as 81 per cent, compared with the 98 per cent for open surgery. This was a big difference, and forced the authors to review whether laparoscopic surgery should be abandoned in favour of the open approach.

In the end they decided that this would be wrong. However, they did suggest that patients should be told beforehand that there might be more complications after 'keyhole' than after open surgery.

At the time of writing this book, five years have passed since their report. Surgeons are now better trained, and have had more experience, in keyhole surgery since the 1990s when the operations in their study were performed. My advice to anyone considering surgery today has two aspects. One is that the Dutch study was in people who had not fully responded to omeprazole, an H^2 antagonist. Today, with most GORD patients on a PPI, I feel that many of them would probably have responded better to their drugs, and so would not have qualified to enter the study in the first place. The second point is that surgeons are now more used to the problems involved in learning keyhole techniques and are more efficient when carrying out keyhole surgery.

GORD patients facing surgery today, therefore, have to weigh up the pros and cons of the two techniques. Open surgery may leave them with a smaller chance of long-term complications, but give them a less comfortable and longer recovery period than keyhole surgery. It is as much up to you, the patient, as it is to the surgeon, as to which type of surgery you opt for. Your surgeon should be able to give the success rates and the complication rates for his or her unit, and to give a comparison with other units. You can then decide together which course you wish to take.

If you are among the 30 per cent or so of GORD sufferers whose problems are linked to a troublesome hiatus hernia, then you may have to face surgery. The next chapter deals with your problem.

9

GORD and hiatus hernia

In medicine, as in many sciences, the pendulum of expert opinion swings to and fro as facts become clear and cherished theories are disproved. Sixty years ago, the experts taught that most people with heartburn had a hiatus hernia. They concluded that if the usual methods of identifying a hernia did not show, they probably were too crude to do so. They accepted, however, that one was probably present.

As X-ray techniques and flexible endoscopy developed and became more sophisticated, they still couldn't find a hiatus hernia in a large proportion of people with GORD, and they had to change their opinion. Not only did they have to accept that acid could flow back up into the oesophagus from the stomach without there being a hernia, there were also times when there was a hernia and no reflux.

More recently, the pendulum has swung back again. The consensus is that hernias underlie many cases of GORD. The problem lies in identifying a small hernia. It certainly is not true that the bigger a hernia, the worse the symptoms are. By 1981, researchers were reporting that around 90 per cent of people with GORD do have small hernias, many of which are missed by the usual hospital techniques. One of the reasons that surgery is so successful in patients with GORD whose symptoms have not responded as well as was hoped to drug treatment, is probably that they have small intermittent hernias that are difficult to spot either on endoscopy or X-ray.

Fundoplication (as described in the last chapter) will automatically repair such hernias, even when they are not seen during actual surgery.

Sliders and rollers

Hiatus hernias occur in two forms: sliders and rollers. Figure 2 shows a sliding hernia. Its basic fault is that the cardia (the junction between the oesophagus and the stomach) is not below the diaphragm, but in the chest. This means that all the mechanisms that prevent the reflux of stomach contents into the oesophagus are lost.

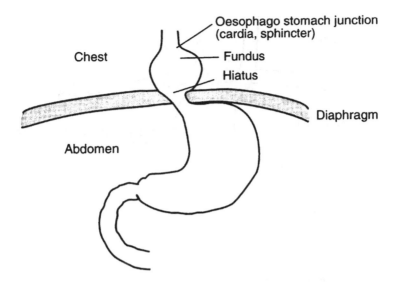

Figure 2 A 'sliding' hernia

As the oesophagus now enters the stomach directly from above, there is no protective 11 o'clock angle or flap valve to prevent upward flow. The crura of the diaphragm no longer encircle the oesophagus, but are loosely arranged around part of the stomach. The sling mechanism to support the 11 o'clock angle is also lost. The part of the stomach that is in the chest freely produces acid and pepsin, and there is no barrier to their flow over the delicate oesophageal lining.

This freedom of flow throughout the oesophagus when there is a sliding hernia is clearly shown if you ask the patient to take two swallows of barium. With the first swallow, some barium collects in the hernial sac above the diaphragm. On the second swallow, when the sphincter (which is of course above the diaphragm) opens to receive the next mouthful, the first lot of barium flows back up the oesophagus. It is clear from this that a small amount of acid is trapped in a hernia at one swallow, and then is ejected up into the oesophagus with the next. This reverse movement only occurs in people with smaller hernias. It does not happen in people with no hernia or with a very large hernia.

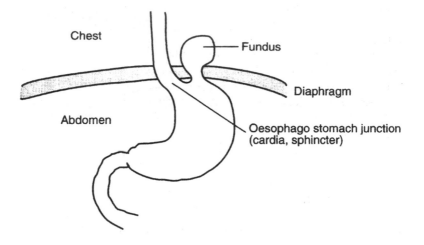

Figure 3   A 'rolling' (para-oesophageal) hernia

The logic of this is odd, but true. Small hernias tend to cause more reflux symptoms than large ones. Yet if you consider the laws of physics, it makes sense. Laplace's law states that the pressure inside a sphere is inversely proportional to its diameter. The larger the hernia, the lower is the pressure inside it. The lower the pressure inside the hernia, the less is the force pushing its contents upwards. If the diameter of the hernia is much greater than that of the oesophagus (a 'balloon hernia') there can be no reflux from the hernial sac into the oesophagus, and usually no heartburn or other symptoms of GORD.

To make things worse, small hernias have narrower outlets, so they retain the pressure inside them for longer; they retain their contents for longer; and the potential for irritation is greater. If the sphincter is relaxed or not working at all, then there will be back-flow up into the oesophagus. In the past, such small hernias were easily missed. Today they may be ignored if their symptoms are kept under control by, say, PPIs.

Only about 5 per cent of hernias are 'rollers'. In rollers the fundus of the stomach 'rolls' up into the chest to lie alongside the lower end of the oesophagus (Figure 3). The cardia remains below the diaphragm and continues to work efficiently. The angle between the lower oesophagus and stomach remains in place, as do the other mechanisms such as the sphincter and the crura. So there should be no reflux with a roller.

However, rollers can give rise to other symptoms. Gas can be trapped in the portion of stomach that lies in the chest, and that causes the bloated feeling that many people describe with it. In contrast with 'sliders', the bigger the roller the more discomfort there is: the only way to get rid of it is to belch and vomit. This can waken people in the night, when they classically roam around the house until the symptoms are relieved. If the roller becomes even bigger, it can take up space normally occupied by your heart and lungs, so that you feel you cannot get a deep breath and your heart can beat erratically.

The main treatment for all rollers, therefore, is surgery to repair the hole in the diaphragm through which it has rolled. Even if the hole is small, an early operation is needed to prevent it from enlarging. It is far better to operate on a hernia under control than to have to do so in an emergency in someone with a blocked loop of stomach or bowel inside a chest in which the heart and lungs are in distress.

So if you present to your doctor with the symptoms of GORD (heartburn and regurgitation) or with deep central bloating and chest pain, his or her thoughts about diagnosis will surely put a hiatus hernia high on the list. But there are other possibilities to be considered. How does your doctor go about sorting them out, one from another? The next chapter is about how your GP tries to do just that.

10

The questions you will be asked

GORD is an unusual medical condition because the GP almost always diagnoses it on the basis of the patient's story alone. The combination of symptoms (heartburn, bloating, regurgitation, acid brash and waterbrash), and the circumstances that bring them on (after meals, bending over, lying down, after putting on weight), make the diagnosis clear. Yet it's natural to have doubts. 'Do I really have this condition?' you may ask yourself.

Shouldn't I have other tests to rule out really nasty illnesses, like cancer or a heart problem? After all, probably the most common health message we hear, time and again, is that a pain in the chest means a heart attack until proved otherwise. And, as many people with GORD find that chest pain is their most troublesome symptom, it is natural that they should be worried about their hearts.

Sometimes these people have been right to worry. Both GORD and heart trouble are common illnesses, and plenty of unlucky people in middle age and beyond develop both. Therefore it is best that they are forewarned about how to tell the difference.

So when you go to your doctor for your first appointment about your symptoms, what can you expect? First of all, a lot of questions!

From what you have read so far – from the case histories, the normal mechanisms of swallowing, the faults that can arise, and the systems we have in place to assess GORD, its severity and how it should be treated – you will understand that you need to describe your symptoms with some accuracy. So prepare yourself beforehand so that you can answer the questions with confidence. Take time to write down your list of symptoms and any questions you may wish to ask.

We will take the usual symptoms of GORD in turn. Try to relate the answers you might give to your doctor with those in each section. We will take heartburn first.

Heartburn

So you have heartburn. Can you describe it in more detail? Is it truly a searing or burning pain, or is it more a dull ache? Exactly where is it? Does it stay behind the breastbone, or does it move up into the jaw or into the left arm? Does it appear in the pit of your stomach, or travel into the back? Does it come on with eating? If so, does the amount or the type of food make a difference?

How you answer these questions will already have narrowed the diagnostic options. The quality of the pain matters a lot. A burning pain points to acid in the oesophagus, a dull ache may mean the development of an oesophageal ulcer, or even pain from the heart (angina). Exactly *where* the pain is also matters. The more widespread it is, the more extensive is the oesophageal irritation, and the more likely it is that you will need more intensive treatment (such as a high dose of a PPI). The burning pain of oesophagitis can extend into the jaw, arm and abdomen, but if your pain is a duller ache in these same areas, your doctor will be thinking of a heart problem, rather than an oesophageal one.

Heartburn with eating, particularly if it comes on immediately you start to eat, is usually from the oesophagus, and the larger the meal, the more likely it is to cause symptoms. However, that is also true of certain types of angina as well, so that the fact that your dull ache is brought on by food does not rule out angina. The interval between starting to eat and the onset of pain, however, is usually longer for angina and for stomach ulcers, another diagnosis likely to be in your doctor's mind.

Oddly, hunger may also bring on heartburn. This does separate it from angina, but not from a stomach ulcer. As for the types of food most likely to bring on heartburn, alcohol, spices, raw fruit, carbonated drinks and hot drinks, especially tea without milk, have topped the list in my experience of listening to patients.

Other pains

Your doctor's next question is likely to be, 'Do you have any other pain, separate from your heartburn?' If you have, try to describe it. What is it like – sharp, dull, intermittent, like cramp? Where is it? What brings it on?

The most common pain for people with GORD, apart from heartburn, is often described as a raw feeling or an aching pain, or just a discomfort that you find very difficult to describe, but is certainly unpleasant, felt mainly in the back of the throat, or in the upper central part of the chest just behind the breastbone. Although it is not usually as severe as heartburn, it is made worse by swallowing food, or hot or cold liquids.

This painful swallowing can be a sign of acute oesophagitis. Regular drinkers (and many people with GORD, I'm afraid, drink too much) will recognize this as the sort of pain they feel in the morning after the 'night before'. Others may feel it after a heavy meal, such as a curry. It does not last long, as acute oesophagitis settles quickly, but it is a warning against future dietary or drinking indiscretions.

A constant ache in the centre of the chest that is not particularly made worse by eating, but may be worse when you are hungry, can be a sign of an ulcer in an irritated oesophagus. It must be taken seriously.

Regurgitation

The second classical symptom of GORD is regurgitation. It is important to get the answer to this one correct when questioned by your GP. Do you find food or drink that you have just swallowed coming back into your mouth? This is different from vomiting, in which you first feel sick, and then the stomach muscles contract to heave the food up from the stomach into the mouth and forcibly outwards. The regurgitation of GORD wells up without any feeling of nausea. Unlike vomiting, you can control the material in your mouth and are not forced to spew it out.

If you do regurgitate, how soon after swallowing does it happen? Does it have the same taste as when it went down, or is there an added sour or bitter taste? Does it arrive with a belch? Do you regurgitate at night, when lying flat? Do you get breathless, and are you prone to chest infections?

The answers to these questions will indicate how serious your problem is, and determine what treatment you should start with (see Chapter 7 for the NICE guidelines on the 'step' treatment schedule). The answers may also decide whether you need to go for further tests. For example, regurgitation immediately after swallowing, combined with the lack of a sour or bitter taste, suggests a blockage in the oesophagus, possibly a stricture from scarring, or achalasia (see page 37). A bitter or sour taste confirms that stomach contents are in the oesophagus, and that there is reflux. Belching is also an indication that stomach contents are involved.

If there is bile – an excessively bitter-tasting green fluid – in the regurgitated material, you also have problems with regurgitation upwards from the duodenum into the stomach. That signals that further tests are essential, in a hurry, as it suggests obstruction further down the gut.

Regurgitation at night also means that you should have further tests. If you regurgitate when asleep, you can inhale some of the material into your lungs. Stomach contents are corrosive and can irritate and damage the lungs. Some American studies have reported that around half of all people with GORD have lung problems such as asthma, bronchitis and bronchiectasis, in which there are multiple pockets of infection deep in the lungs. They have not been confirmed by Europeans, and there is still argument about the proportion of people with GORD who inhale regurgitated materials when asleep. However, if you do find your mouth filling up with fluid when lying flat, you should ask your doctor about surgery. Correcting reflux with surgery (see Chapter 8) has been reported not just to cure the symptoms of GORD, but also, where people have had chest problems, to cure them too.

'Sticking'

Let's take swallowing in more detail. Do you have difficulty in swallowing? Does it feel as if food sticks inside your chest? How often does this happen? Is it getting worse?

The feeling that food isn't slipping down as easily as it should is common in GORD. It can mean one of two problems. When it 'comes and goes', it is usually a sign of oesophagitis – irritation of the oesophagus due to acid regurgitation. When you are given drugs such as a PPI to remove the acid, the condition quickly improves, and the feeling disappears.

However, if the feeling of food 'sticking' is getting worse, happening more often, and especially after each meal, then your doctor will suspect a stricture. Strictures are fixed narrowed scars that are usually the end-result of many episodes of oesophagitis. Repeated inflammation and healing eventually produces scars that contract and constrict the diameter of the oesophagus. They do not open up, even under pressure. They can form at any level in the oesophagus.

Some swallowing problems are caused by spasm of the oesophagus, such as the achalasia and nutcracker oesophagus described in

Chapter 3. They also give the feeling that food is held up deep inside the chest, but their main symptom is pain, and the feeling suddenly disappears along with the pain as the cramp eases off. However, in more severe forms of achalasia the symptoms are so like a stricture that endoscopy is needed to tell the difference.

Feeling that food 'sticks' and that you have difficulty in swallowing ('dysphagia') is so important that I've devoted the next chapter to it. If you recognize these features as part of your symptoms of GORD, please read it.

Stooping and bending

Do your symptoms get worse when you adopt a particular posture – for example, when you are stooping, bending over, lying down? Do they come on when you are lifting heavy weights? How comfortable are you in bed? Do you have to sleep propped up? Are you woken up at night with heartburn?

If your GORD is due to a sliding hernia, your symptoms are likely to be greatly influenced by the position you adopt. If the pain starts when you stoop, bend or lie down, you probably have a 'slider' with reflux. The symptoms are often worst in bed, and many people have discovered, long before they finally seek their doctor's advice, that sleeping propped up on several pillows eases their symptoms.

I'll return here to the advice (given by the GP guidelines listed on p. 49) about putting blocks under the head of the bed. I've found that if that's all that you do, you end up sliding down the bed when you fall asleep, and end up horizontal anyway. One way to deal with that is to put a blocking board in the foot of the bed, so that your feet come up against it, to prevent you from sliding down any further. Better still, put blocks under the *foot* of the bed, and an angled support under your pillows. This will prop your torso up at an angle of around 60 degrees, and your legs will also be propped up at an angle of around 10 degrees. Then any tendency to slide when you fall asleep will be towards the head of your bed, reinforcing the desired angle, instead of reducing it. This should keep you relatively upright when asleep.

Belching and bloating

Do you belch a lot? Do you feel bloated? How often does it happen? It is embarrassing to belch and to feel bloated, but you can be reassured that these symptoms are not signs of serious disease. Some people feel so bloated that they worry that their abdomen might burst. It won't.

If you are badly affected by constant 'wind', you may not like what you read here, but it's true. Most excessive belching is caused by you swallowing excessive amounts of air. The process is an unconscious one, so don't blame yourself for it. Everyone swallows a little air from time to time, but 'big belchers' swallow every few seconds. When they do so, down goes a little saliva and a lot of air. This air has to be belched up or passed on into the gut from the stomach, where it must eventually reach the other end of the digestive system.

Your answer is to try to stop air-swallowing. That's more difficult to do than it seems, because once you know you have a habit, it can be even more intense. You may need training in relaxation to help yourself. Your doctor or one of the nursing staff at the surgery may be trained in relaxation, or may know someone who could help.

Everyone has some gas in the stomach. It is a normal part of digestion, and some air has to be swallowed to keep the contents of the bowel flowing. If you have a rolling hiatus hernia, however, the air can gather in the fundus and be trapped there. It then causes pain and discomfort deep inside the chest. The trick is to find out how best to displace the air back into the part of the stomach that remains inside the abdomen, and then belch it up. Some people do it by getting up and roaming around the house in the middle of the night, others find lying on one side helps. Many find an antacid-alginate medicine eases the gas discomfort.

However, if you find that you are constantly belching and bloated, you must tell your doctor. They are a classical sign of a rolling hernia that needs an operation to replace the fundus under the diaphragm (see page 70). Rolling hernias have a habit of enlarging quickly, and you definitely do not want to wait until you are in an emergency.

Bleeding

Your doctor will also ask about bleeding. Have you noticed any flecks of blood in the material you have regurgitated? What colour are your stools? Have they ever been black?

Acid reflux can cause small blood vessels in the lining of the oesophagus to erode, leading to bleeding, which you will see as flecks of red or rusty brown in the liquid that appears in your mouth. However, if you don't regurgitate, and your only symptom is heartburn, you may be bleeding without knowing it. The only way to be sure is to examine your stools. By the time blood has travelled from the oesophagus to the anus it is changed chemically, so that it is now black, rather than red. A stool containing a lot of blood also changes in consistency, so that it is like passing soft tar. If this happens, you must see your doctor immediately, as black tarry stools ('melaena') are a reason for emergency admission to hospital, so that the bleeding can be stopped and you can be transfused if necessary. Absolutely do not ignore melaena: it can be fatal if you don't seek urgent help.

Melaena is a relatively rare complication of GORD. The blood loss from a chronically irritated oesophagus can be only a few millilitres a day. There is not enough to show obviously in the stools: they may be a little darker brown than normal, but you will probably not notice the change. The stools remain normally formed. However, even the loss of 3 or 4 ml a day over many months can be enough to cause anaemia.

Even though the stools look normal, the modern tests for blood in them will easily detect such small amounts. When you see your doctor for your GORD symptoms, you will probably be asked to give a sample of your blood for a haemoglobin test. If it shows that you are anaemic, don't be surprised if your doctor asks for a stool sample. It is usual practice to ask for three specimens taken on successive days. If you have blood in the stools and are anaemic, then you will almost certainly be asked to see a specialist.

Very occasionally oesophagitis causes no symptoms, and the first sign of trouble is a haemorrhage, which can rise into the mouth or be passed through the anus as melaena. This is sometimes an indication of a Barrett's oesophagus (see p. 35), in which the changes in the cells lining the oesophagus makes them less sensitive to painful stimuli such as acid. If you have this problem, it's likely you will be asked to undergo surgery to remove the ulcerated area. You will then be put on lifelong PPI treatment to try to prevent a recurrence.

Coughing

Several times in this book I've referred to people with GORD who become 'chesty'. They get lung complications because they have acid in their oesophagus – but do they have to inhale this acid to become chesty? That's a subject that the experts have been arguing about for years. Some people with GORD have a permanent hoarseness, apparently because their voice box (larynx) is irritated by the reflux. Others have GORD-related asthma which can present as a wheeze or a chronic cough. Yet others develop pneumonia and lung abscesses. These are serious, sometimes life-threatening conditions. If you are affected by them, you need very careful and comprehensive treatment.

The connection between GORD and chest problems is not a simple one. In studies of more than 4,000 scans of people with GORD who were asked to swallow, only 2 per cent actually breathed in their refluxed stomach contents. This was completely contradicted by a study in only 19 people who were scanned overnight when asleep. Five of them inhaled their stomach contents when asleep.

So at least some of the chesty symptoms may be due to inhaling refluxed stomach contents. But there is another possible explanation. The vagus nerve (which among other activities helps to control the heartbeat and to narrow the airways) directly connects the oesophagus and the bronchi – the main airways to the lungs. Put a little acid into the lower end of the oesophagus of a susceptible patient and the bronchi will immediately narrow, producing a wheeze. There is no need for the patient to inhale any acid: the presence of the acid in the oesophagus is enough to set off the reaction, presumably through stimulating the vagus nerve.

Children seem to be particularly susceptible to wheeze when acid enters the lower oesophagus. In a study of 20 children with asthma monitored overnight, their attacks were associated with acid entering the oesophagus through a hiatus hernia. When their hiatus hernias were repaired at operation, both the symptoms of their oesophagitis and their chest problems disappeared. In another study, when cimetidine was given to children with reflux-induced asthma, their asthma improved. The same may well be true of many adults. PPIs should work even more effectively for them.

Cancer

I've left the question of cancer to the last section of this chapter because that's the place patients usually put it. It is what they really are worried about, but can't pluck up the courage to bring up the subject. So they talk about everything else until they have their hand on the doorknob on the way out. Then it starts with 'Oh, and by the way, Doctor . . .'

As doctors, we learn very early that the 'hand on doorknob' question is always the one that the patient really wanted to discuss throughout the consultation. So we sit back, invite the patient back to his or her seat, and start again. To give people their due, today fewer people are reticent about the subject than in the previous generation, and that's a good sign. In these days of openness and frankness about medical conditions, it is vital that you should have a heightened suspicion when the symptoms change or something, perhaps indefinable, is not right.

It is natural for people who have difficulty in swallowing, regurgitation and central chest pain to think of cancer. Cancers do occur in the oesophagus, and may or may not be linked with years of reflux disease. Their main symptom is difficulty in swallowing. It is unusual for cancers to cause heartburn or pain. The first symptom may arise out of the blue, perhaps when trying to swallow a larger piece of food than usual, such as a piece of meat that you have not thoroughly chewed. Or it may develop gradually, so that swallowing becomes slower and the food seems to take longer to 'go down' than it used to. In later stages of oesophageal cancer you lose the pleasure in eating and drinking, and shed weight because you are not eating.

However, you should have gone to your doctor long before you reached that stage. Anyone with difficulty in swallowing should always see his or her doctor, who will always refer the case to a specialist for endoscopy and perhaps a scan during swallowing. Most of the time, and especially when there are other GORD symptoms such as heartburn, the trouble turns out to be caused by a stricture. This is scarring and narrowing because of years of exposure to refluxed acid and pepsin.

A relatively rare cause of swallowing difficulties has three names. Its basic name is sideropaenic dysphagia. Doctors call it Patterson-Brown-Kelly syndrome or Plummer-Vinson syndrome, depending on the medical school that trained them. It affects women between

30 and 60 and has three features: severe anaemia, chronic inflammation of the tongue, and choking when trying to swallow solids.

Affected women initially have muscle spasms in the upper half of the oesophagus, which eventually lead to a stricture that makes the swallowing difficulty much worse. A 'web' of thin tissue forms across the top of the larynx which, if neglected and not removed, can become cancerous. The treatment is to give iron to reverse the anaemia and to remove the stricture at operation.

Cancer of the oesophagus is a disease of older age: 75 per cent of cases are in people over 60 years old. It affects three times more men than women. About half of all oesophageal cancers arise in its middle third and about 30 per cent in its lower third. Oddly, this distribution of cancers suggests to the experts that they are linked to acid reflux. Although the lower third is more exposed to acid, the middle third is thought to be more sensitive to acid-provoked cancerous changes.

Stopping GORD in its tracks by PPI treatment and preventing acid reaching the oesophagus may therefore prevent many cancers, which is a good reason for you to stick to your doctor's advice on how to manage GORD. This is particularly true of Barrett's oesophagus, which carries a higher than usual risk of cancerous change (see p. 36).

As long ago as 1985, before PPIs were invented, R. Kuylenstierna and E. Munch-Wickland, writing in the *Journal of Cancer*, looked back on the cases of 163 patients with oesophageal cancer. Of the 51 patients with cancer in the lower third of the oesophagus, 25 per cent had had oesophagitis. Of the 47 with cancer of the upper third, none had had it. They concluded that chronic oesophagitis can precede cancer of the lower oesophagus if reflux is not controlled or eradicated.

So you have an extra motive for seeking a cure for your GORD. Not only will it ease your symptoms, it should also offer some protection against oesophageal cancer.

11

Dysphagia – when food 'sticks'

One consequence of years of heartburn is that the oesophagus may become scarred and narrowed. The normal muscular control of swallowing described in Chapter 2 can be disturbed, so that solid foods become 'stuck' at the point where the oesophagus is narrowed, and even thick liquids can be held up on their way down towards the stomach.

This is 'dysphagia'. It is a severe symptom, and is one of the 'alarm' symptoms described in Chapter 4 that will make your GP send you urgently for a specialist opinion. There is good reason for this: dysphagia may be just the sign of scarring or spasm of the oesophagus ('achalasia'), but it may also be an early sign of cancer of the oesophagus, and that must be ruled out (usually by endoscopy) before it can be dealt with properly.

If you do have a cancer, then much can be done, from removing the tumour-bearing area of oesophagus, to radiotherapy or chemo-therapy, or inserting a 'stent' that bypasses the constriction and allows you to swallow again.

Most people with dysphagia, however, do not have cancer: their swallowing difficulties are entirely due to their GORD. The oesophagitis has caused scarring or oesophageal muscle spasm. Even if cancer has been ruled out, you still have to deal with the problem – and that can be severe. Being unable to eat properly undermines your confidence and your dignity, so that you stop eating with others. It destroys your social life and isolates you from family and friends. Not only that, you tend to stop trying to eat, so that you are slowly starving yourself. Along with losing your enjoyment in eating, you shed weight and you lose your fitness.

Strangely, the British seem to fare worse than other Europeans when it comes to coping with dysphagia. In one survey of 360 patients with dysphagia in four European countries,[9] including the UK, 44 per cent of them had lost weight; 60 per cent were eating too little; 59 per cent still felt hungry after their mealtimes; 73 per cent stated that they no longer enjoyed life because of their eating problems; 68 per cent were embarrassed by their problems; and 36 per cent now ate alone, being too embarrassed to dine with others.

Sadly, only 33 per cent were receiving professional treatment for their dysphagia.

Dysphagia can put you at real risk of malnutrition, so that you become progressively weaker, more prone to infections, exhausted, and tired all the time. You can't enjoy the company of friends and family, and many people with swallowing difficulties become almost hermits, living and eating alone. It's not surprising that depression is a major problem for them.

The main problem in dysphagia is with solid or semi-solid foods. However, most people with it tend not to drink enough, either. Although they can swallow fluids, even that can be a bother, so they tend to ignore their thirst, and shy away from drinking as well as eating. If you are at that stage, please heed the next few paragraphs.

If you are having swallowing difficulties you absolutely must drink enough to keep you well hydrated. Your body needs the fluids. One of the first symptoms of dehydration is a dry mouth, with too little saliva. That makes it even more difficult to swallow, and it also changes the environment for the bacteria in the mouth, making it easier to develop a mouth infection. So the first priority is to keep drinking plenty of watery fluids.

If you are finding it really difficult to swallow, and meals take much longer than they should, then take advice from your doctor on how to cope better. If you can, liquidize your food, so that it can slip down with minimum effort on your part. Make sure that the food is still tasty, though, because there is nothing more likely to put you off liquidized meals than bland pap. Eat small meals often, rather than your usual three meals a day. If you have been losing weight, ask your doctor about adding protein and energy-rich drinks to your daily intake of food. They can be prescribed on the NHS for people with swallowing problems.

You probably have a preference for either sweet or savoury foods – make sure that you get what you want. There are prepared foods that suit the tastes of most people.

Check that your teeth and gums are in good order: if you wear dentures, they should be good working teeth, not for show, as so many are. I'm often surprised by the people who have to take their teeth out to eat.

Finally, if your dysphagia is dominating your life, there are several ways to help. Specialists in oesophageal surgery can widen any narrowing using a series of dilators, or 'bougies', passed under local anaesthetic while you are under sedation. You may need a more complex operation involving re-shaping the oesophagus, perhaps by bringing up a loop of small intestine from the abdomen to replace the narrowed area. In extreme cases, nutrition can be given via a tube in the abdomen, direct into the stomach. However, that is very much a last resort to save a life. Such surgery was more common in times when we had few effective medical treatments: today, many GPs have never had to care for a patient who has needed this type of surgery.

12

Could it really be my heart?
Checking out your chest pain

Having read this far, you know by now that one of the main features
of GORD is pain in the chest. The pain may not be just heartburn –
which most people recognize and appreciate is related to digestion.
GORD also produces a deep pain in the chest that can be described
as an ache or a boring pain, that can also radiate into the back and
side. As explained in a previous chapter, this may be caused by
spasm of the oesophagus or by ulcers in an irritated oesophagus,
such as a Barrett's oesophagus. Doctors like myself often find it
difficult to differentiate between this sort of pain and the pain due to
angina pectoris – pain due to heart disease. If we find it difficult, it's
not surprising that you, the person with the pain, also find it
worrying.

So how can you reassure yourself that the pain you are
experiencing is not angina? I'll start to answer that with a definition.
Angina is simply the medical word for pain. Angina pectoris means
pain in the chest, but the two words together have become, in
common usage, synonymous with heart pain.

However, many pains in the chest have no connection with the
heart. For example, injuries to, or inflammation in, the spine, ribs
and chest muscles can lead to persistent pain that can frighten you
into believing you are having a heart attack. Nerve irritations from
shingles can mimic angina. Pleurisy, an inflammation or infection of
the lung surface, can cause severe chest pains, and we have already
covered in a previous chapter the chest pains that GORD can cause.

So if your main complaint is chest pain, your doctor will ask
searching questions about it, and your answers will narrow down the
possible causes.

What is the pain like?

The first will be about the character of the pain. Can you describe
exactly what it feels like in simple terms? The ways in which heart

pain affects you are well defined. If you describe it in the following ways, your doctor's suspicions will be aroused:

- Tightness across my chest.
- A weight or pressure on my chest.
- Constriction in my chest.
- An aching pain.
- A dull ache.
- A squeezing feeling.
- It's just sore.
- My chest is being crushed.
- There's a band around my chest.
- The tightness makes me breathless.

If the pain is more like the list below, your doctor will be looking for another cause, such as GORD or chest muscle problems:

- It's sharp.
- It's like a knife cutting into me.
- It comes in stabs, like colic.
- It feels like a stitch.
- It's like needles in my skin.
- It shoots across my chest.
- It's worse when you press on it.
- It's worse when I change position.
- I can walk around all day with it.
- It's there all day, even when I'm resting.

Where is the pain?

The next question is about where the pain is. Heart pain tends to be on the left side, and it can spread into the jaw, down into the left arm, into the back and even into the upper stomach. It can feel as if it is vaguely in the centre of the chest, but most people with angina identify it as more on the left than the exact centre. It is very rare for it to be entirely right-sided. An entirely right-sided pain is hardly ever due to heart problems, except in the very rare case (fewer than 1 in 10,000) of a 'mirror-image' twin in whom all the organs are reversed, with the heart on the right, and liver and appendix on the left. I had a good friend, Ken, with this condition. He was regularly asked to appear at medical school final examinations, to try to catch out the students on their chest examinations. If the students were nice to him he would whisper the diagnosis to them as they bent over him, puzzled at not finding the heartbeat on his left side.

Oesophageal pain is almost always central, with no bias to left or right.

What brings the pain on?

The third question is – when does the pain arise? Most heart pain starts with exercise. Physical effort brings it on, and resting relieves it. The more strenuous the exercise is, the more likely you are to develop the pain. When you stop, the pain stops as the strain on the heart falls away. Oesophageal pain is related to food and perhaps to hunger, but not to exercise. It is eased by antacids: heart pain is not.

One problem with this is that eating can induce angina, as the effort of chewing, swallowing and digesting the food makes the heart work harder: if it is prone to angina, eating can bring it on. So not all pain that arises with eating is necessarily due to GORD. If one of your GORD symptoms has been pain with eating, you will know from experience what that feels like. It will differ in quality from an anginal pain, so be wary of any pain in the chest that has a new character to it, or is in a slightly different place, and doesn't go away with your usual antacid preparation. Angina is such a common illness that it's quite possible to have both GORD and heart problems. Make sure that you ask your doctor's advice if you develop a new type of chest pain that you feel isn't quite your usual sort.

How do you cope with the pain?

The final question is – what do you do when the pain starts? Do you have to stop and rest to make it disappear? Or can you keep on doing what you have been doing, such as walking? If it tends to disappear while you are still exercising, it is unlikely to be angina. If you absolutely *must* rest to relieve the pain, it is almost certainly a heart problem.

There is good reason for this. The heart obeys a law as

87

fundamental in biology as it is in the marketplace – supply and demand. The supply is the blood in the coronary arteries carrying oxygen and glucose to fuel the beating of the heart muscle. The demand comes from the need for the heart muscle to beat so that it can supply blood to all the other organs and tissues. The more energy we expend in exercise, in digesting food or even in solving an intellectual problem, the more blood the heart needs to pump to the muscles, gut and brain. To do this, the heart itself needs more blood, supplied through the coronary arteries, to deal with the higher work rate of its muscle. The coronary arteries must open up to deal with the greater flow of blood. If they can't open sufficiently, the heart can't get enough oxygen to feed its blood to its muscle. This leads to a build-up of waste products in the heart muscle, which we feel as pain. When we rest, the heart returns to its normal working pattern, the waste products are flushed away, and the pain recedes.

If you want to know more about heart problems leading to angina, please read my book *Heart Attacks – Prevent and Survive* (also published by Sheldon Press). I mention heart pain here for two reasons – to reassure you that the pains of GORD and of angina are usually very different, and to guide you when you think that you may have angina alongside your GORD. If, having read these last few pages, you still wonder if your pain may be a heart problem, then see your doctor.

13
The ongoing debate – whom to investigate?

I described in Chapter 4 the guidelines on treatment of dyspepsia (which includes GORD) that NICE has laid down for GPs to follow. They can be summarized as follows:

- People with alarm symptoms such as dysphagia (see Chapter 10) or weight loss, at any age, should be sent for endoscopy.
- People without alarm symptoms, but who are presumed to have GORD, should be treated first according to the 'step' system (see p. 61) without the need for endoscopy.
- People over 55 years old who have GORD symptoms for the first time should be treated first, and sent for endoscopy only if the treatment does not help.

The aim of these guidelines was to reduce the very high demand for endoscopy. GPs in the UK have 'open access' to endoscopy services. That is, they can order endoscopies for their patients without first having to refer them to a specialist. Since this scheme started, endoscopy services have become in danger of being overwhelmed by requests for appointments for patients whose symptoms were not in the 'alarm' category, and who turned out to have simple, uncomplicated GORD. This was leading to longer waiting times, with possibly fatal consequences for the minority of patients who had serious illness. That was the main reason for the advice that people over 55 with a provisional diagnosis of GORD should first have a trial of treatment before having an endoscopy.

In 2005, delegates at the British Society of Gastroenterology Conference argued strongly against the NICE guidelines. The disagreement arose from a study led by Dr Andrew Goddard, consultant gastroenterologist at Derby City Hospital. He and his colleagues suggested that patients' lives were being put at risk by the NICE guidelines. They argued that if they delayed endoscopy in older patients with new symptoms not in the alarm category until after they had a test treatment period, they would miss a substantial number of people with early cancer. By the time these patients had their endoscopies, their cancers might have moved from a curable to a non-curable stage.

In their study of 480 patients, they said, 1 in 15 patients referred over the age of 55 with new-onset dyspepsia and no alarm symptoms turned out to have cancer. Dr Goddard was therefore 'very uncomfortable' with delaying diagnosis by the three months it would take to follow the 'treat first' system. He asked that endoscopy must not be delayed by symptomatic treatments, and wanted to use his results to persuade GPs to ignore the NICE advice on older patients.

He wasn't alone. One of his colleagues in the research, Professor Michael Griffen, president of the Association of Upper Gastrointestinal Surgeons of Great Britain and Ireland, insisted at the same meeting that the NICE guidance was 'absolute nonsense'. He said that they would not pick up patients who are potentially curable, and that struck him as 'fundamentally flawed'. In the study, cancer was found in 7 per cent of those with no alarm symptoms, 7 per cent of those with one alarm symptom, and 16 per cent of those with two alarm symptoms.

Dr David Lyon, of Halton, a GP with a special interest in cancer diagnosis and management, agreed that if GPs knew that 1 in 15 people with new-onset dyspepsia has cancer, they would refer for endoscopy straight away. He has a strong point.

On the other side of this argument stands Dr Mark Follows. He is an unusual doctor, who spent three years as a registrar in gastroenterology before becoming a GP. He still spends three working sessions a week in GP-oriented gastroenterology, and one of his tasks is to implement the NICE guidelines among the doctors in his region of West Yorkshire.

While he was still a hospital specialist, Dr Follows was involved in a review of 1,000 GP-instituted open access endoscopies for dyspepsia. They revealed only seventeen cancers, nine in the oesophagus and eight in the stomach. All had had 'alarm symptoms'. The nine with oesophageal cancer had dysphagia: the eight with gastric cancer had either lost weight or had anaemia, or both. Not one cancer was found among the others with no alarm symptoms. Dr Follows writes:[10] 'The holy grail of open-access endoscopy was to find early treatable upper GI [gastrointestinal] cancers and it simply has not done that.'

Dr Follows has backed up this view with a further study. He has reviewed, in 2005, 240 fast-track referrals to his local general hospital unit in Airedale, Yorkshire. These patients were fast-tracked because they had at least one alarm symptom or there were other reasons for urgent tests. Even in those with alarm symptoms, only 1 in 10 had a serious disease such as ulcers, and only 1 in 20 had cancer.

He stresses that the new NICE guidelines had been 'distilled out of years of work in this area by the Cochrane group' and, unlike the study by Dr Goddard and his colleagues, was not based on just one group of 480 patients. The Cochrane group is a worldwide network of co-operating reviewers of scientific papers on medical trials, hugely respected for its integrity, its objectivity and its accuracy. Its findings are the gold standard for all medical research today.

So where does that leave me, as a doctor, when faced with a patient, possibly like yourself, who comes to me with new symptoms of GORD, and who is 55 or older? Do I ask for an endoscopy, or do I treat and hope? Will you be satisfied with treat and hope, or will you want to demand an endoscopy to make sure that you are not seriously ill, say, with cancer?

On balance, I'm inclined to side with Dr Follows and NICE. I'd treat first, using the 'step' method and advice on lifestyle, and expect the vast majority of you to get better very quickly. If there were no response within, say, three to four weeks, however, I would not wait three months, but discuss your case with the local consultant gastroenterologist, usually by phone. We are blessed in our region (the west of Scotland) with excellent relationships between GPs and consultants, so we can do that quickly and efficiently. Whenever I have done this, the consultant has usually either suggested different treatment for perhaps two weeks more, or has gone straight to endoscopy. The decision to turn earlier or later to endoscopy depends on the history of the symptoms, their character, their duration, their response to treatment and the patient's age. The length of the endoscopy waiting list, and where the patient might lie in order of priority on it, also matters.

So should you, as a patient, push for earlier investigation because you fear that your symptoms are suspicious? If everyone acted in that way, waiting lists would lengthen, and people whose need for an endoscopy is greater than yours may miss out. Delay may be lethal for them, but only an inconvenience for you. I leave it to you to decide. If you have no alarm symptoms, I don't think you have a case for pushing for endoscopy, but if your GORD symptoms persist despite going through the 'step' method, then you should have an endoscopy. If you have one or more alarm symptoms, at any age, then I'd send you for an open access endoscopy as a first step, while starting treatment without delay.

Conclusion

Now you know all about GORD! I hope this book will help you to take action in areas where it may be needed – most importantly, losing weight, drinking less, and giving up smoking. I also hope that what I've written will take you to your doctor when necessary. If in doubt, do go. As you saw from the case histories in Chapter 1, reflux and heartburn present and develop in many different ways and at many different stages of life, and in other chapters I've also described how GORD can sometimes coexist with other conditions.

So, if in doubt, do get yourself checked out. There are plenty of effective treatments to minimize the symptoms, to help heal the oesophageal irritation, and make life more comfortable while you focus on more long-term lifestyle changes that will also help your GORD. And remember, you may need your doctor to help you differentiate between the subtle changes in symptoms when an apparent bout of reflux symptoms is in fact a bout of angina, or other heart trouble. Meanwhile, I hope you will take comfort from the fact that your GORD is to a large extent in your own hands, and that the choices you start making from today can make a real difference.

References

1 M. Ruth, I. Manson and N. Sandberg, 'The prevalence of symptoms suggestive of oesophageal disorders', *Scandinavian Journal of Gastroenterology*, 26, 1991, pp. 73–81.

2 E. Dimenas, 'Methodological aspects of evaluation of quality of life in upper gastrointestinal disease', *Scandinavian Journal of Gastroenterology*, 28 (supplement 199), 1993, pp. 18–21.

3 D. A. Revicki, M. Wood, P. N. Maton *et al.*, 'The impact of gastroesophageal reflux disease on health-related quality of life', *American Journal of Medicine*, 104, 1998, pp. 252–8.

4 J. Dent, R. Jones, P. Kahrilas and N. J. Tadley, 'Management of gastro-oesophageal reflux disease in general practice', *British Medical Journal*, 322, 2001, pp. 344–7.

5 J. Dent, J. Brun, A. M. Fendrick *et al.*, 'An evidence-based appraisal of reflux disease management – the Genval workshop report', *Gut*, 44 (supplement 2), 1999, S1–S16.

6 L. Lundell, P. Miettinen and H. E. Myrvold *et al.*, 'Long-term management of gastro-oesophageal reflux disease with omeprazole or open anti-reflux surgery: results of a prospective randomized clinical trial', *European Journal of Gastroenterology and Hepatology*, 12, 2000, pp. 879–87.

7 B. Dallemagne, J. M. Weerts and Jehaes *et al.*, 'Laparoscopic Nissen fundoplication: preliminary report', *Surgical Laparoscopic Endoscopy*, 1, 1991, pp. 138–43.

8 J. E. Bais, J. F. W. M. Bartelsman, H. J. Bonjer *et al.*, 'Laparoscopic or conventional Nissen fundoplication for gastro-oesophageal reflux disease: randomised clinical trial', *Lancet*, 335, 2000, pp. 170–4.

9 O. Ekberg *et al.*, 'A European survey assessing the impact of dysphagia', European Study Group for Diagnosis and Therapy of Dysphagia and Globus, 1999.

10 M. Follows, 'Failures of open-access endoscopy', *Pulse*, 65, issue 12 (26 March), 2005, p. 31.

Index